OPTOMETRY
EDITION 2.1

ROGER F. FILIPS, OD, FAAO

VALERIE M. KATTOUF, OD, FAAO

Reviewers
David J. Dawson, OD
Cynthia G. Heard, OD

First Edition Reviewers
Kevin T. Corcoran, OD
Karl C. Golnik, MD
Gregory A. Kiracofe, OD, FAAO
Susan McCollough, MD
Michael E. Snyder, MD

Resident Reviewers
Michael Dobos, OD, MS
John P. Maszczak, OD
Priscilla R. Schaeffer, OD
J. Erin Shewring, OD
Kelly Thompson, OD

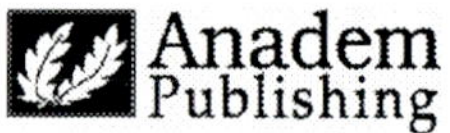

Anadem
Publishing
Anadem Publishing, Inc.
3620 North High Street
Columbus, OH 43214
Tel: 1 (800) 633-0055
www.anadem.com

Clinical Pearls for Optometry, Ed. 2.1

By
Roger F. Filips, OD, FAAO
Valerie M. Kattouf, OD, FAAO

Reviewers
David J. Dawson, OD
Cynthia G. Heard, OD

First Edition Reviewers
Kevin T. Corcoran, OD
Karl C. Golnik, MD
Gregory A. Kiracofe, OD, FAAO
Susan McCollough, MD
Michael E. Snyder, MD

Resident Reviewers
Michael Dobos, OD, MS
John P. Maszczak, OD
Priscilla R. Schaeffer, OD
J. Erin Shewring, OD
Kelly Thompson, OD

ISBN 1-890018-68-6

Acknowledgments

While none of us can name all of the instructors and mentors who have formed our clinical skills, there are a few world-class clinicians whose knowledge and experience comprise much of what is condensed in this book.

Greg Kiracofe	Chief of Optometry, Dayton VAMC
Kevin Corcoran	Director of Optometric Services, Cincinnati Eye Institute
Richard Kerstine	Vitreous, Cincinnati Eye Institute
Linda Greff	Glaucoma, Cincinnati Eye Institute
Adam Kaufman	Uveitis, Cincinnati Eye Institute
Robert Foster	Retina and Vitreous, Cincinnati Eye Institute
Michael Snyder	Anterior Segment, Cincinnati Eye Institute
Karl Golnik	Neuro-ophthalmology, Cincinnati Eye Institute
Gary Varley	Anterior Segment, Cincinnati Eye Institute
Susan McCollough	Emergency Department, Fairmont Medical Center, Mayo Health Systems

I also need to thank my reviewers, Greg Kiracofe, Kevin Corcoran, Michael Snyder, Karl Golnik and Susan McCollough. Thank you to my family for the time I took from you to write this.

Using This Book

Publisher's Note

Clinical Pearls for Optometry — is based upon information from sources believed to be reliable. In developing this book the publisher, authors, contributors, reviewers, and editors have made substantial efforts to make sure that the regimens, drugs, and treatments are correct and are in accordance with currently accepted standards. Readers are cautioned to use their own judgment in making clinical decisions and, when appropriate, consult and compare information from other resources since ongoing research and clinical experience yield new information and since there is the possibility of human error in developing a resource such as this. Attention should be paid to checking the product information supplied by drug manufacturers when prescribing or administering drugs. The publisher, author, reviewers, contributors, and editors disclaim any liability, loss or damage as result, directly or indirectly, from using or applying any of the contents of this book.

FOREWORD

There are some new people to thank who have pitched in to make this second edition of *Clinical Pearls* bigger and better than the first.

First of all I thank Valerie Kattouf from the Illinois College of Optometry for taking time to write the new chapters on pediatric examination and vision training. This makes *Clinical Pearls* the total optometric pocket reference, covering everything from accommodative problems to zoster, herpes.

I also need to thank David Dawson and Cynthia Heard from The Ohio State University College of Optometry for their knowledge and painstakingly detailed proofreading. The book is better and more professional for their efforts.

I also thank you, the purchaser of *Clinical Pearls*. If you use this book to better care for one of your patients, it makes it all worthwhile.

Roger F. Filips, OD, FAAO
Filips Eye Clinic, Hartington NE
Clinical Instructor, The Ohio State University College of Optometry
Consulting Optometrist, Dayton VAMC

TABLE OF CONTENTS

1

TOPICAL OCULAR MEDICATIONS

Stick to what works best; avoid obsolete drugs.

A) Antibiotic drops
1) Polytrim 10 mL: for mild to moderate bacterial infections: effective, inexpensive, generic
2) Vigamox 3 mL, Zymar 5 mL: 4th generation fluoroquinolone, most effective topical antibiotics for severe infections (although only labeled for conjunctivitis so far)

B) Antibiotic ointment
1) Bacitracin: for all abrasions, lid margin staph, and any chronic use
2) Polysporin: for acute use, broader spectrum but may get toxic reaction with long term use
3) Ciloxan: for serious pediatric bacterial infections when frequent drop instillation is a problem

C) Antivirals
1) Viroptic 7.5 mL: for herpes simplex keratitis

D) Steroid drops
1) FML 1, 5, 10, 15 mL: episcleritis, epidemic keratoconjunctivitis, allergies, etc.
2) Pred Forte 1, 5, 10, 15 mL: for all iritis: most likely to cause posterior subcapsular cataracts and intraocular pressure (IOP) rise with long term use. Do not substitute generic if bad inflammation
3) Lotemax 2.5, 5, 10 mL: less IOP rise than Pred Forte, but use 1½ – 2x the dosing. Do not use for acute iritis

E) Antibiotic steroid combination drops
1) Tobradex 2.5, 5, 10 mL: combination tobramycin and 0.1% dexamethasone. Convenient combination treatment of staph marginal infiltrates

2) Zylet 2.5, 5, 10 mL: combination tobramycin and loteprednol for more safety and steroid potency

F) Antibiotic/steroid ointment
1) Tobradex ointment: convenient treatment of inflammatory blepharitis

G) Topical analgesia
1) Voltaren 2.5 or 5 mL or Nevanac 3 mL: NSAID pain reduction
2) Proparacaine 0.5% 15 mL or tetracaine 0.5% 15 mL for short term topical anesthesia for most topical procedures
3) Lidocaine 4% used topically is the most effective drop for painful procedures. Use with 2.5% phenylephrine to increase duration

H) Non-preserved bottled artificial tears: Gen Teal, Refresh Tears, Refresh Liquigel, Systane, Optive
1) Do not cause preservative sensitivity
2) Are less expensive and more convenient than single dose drops
3) Use if will need chronic dosing >four times per day (qid), will save having to sort out a worsening dry eye vs. preservative sensitivity later
4) All other tears can be used for less frequent dosing. There is little clinical difference
5) Restasis (cyclosporine 0.05%): an immunomodulator eye drop to treat many of the underlying inflammatory causes of dry eye. Topical steroids such as Lotemax are also helpful (very expensive and improvement takes months)

I) Anti-rosacea: MetroGel, MetroCream or MetroLotion
1) Labeled to apply to affected skin, not eyes
2) Published evidence that it works on ocular rosacea also, with no side effects

J) Anti-allergy drops
1) Mild to moderate symptoms (Sx): Similasan Allergy Eye Relief 10 mL tid – qid, works well instilled while wearing contacts (unlabeled use)
2) Acute Sx: Naphcon A 15 mL or equivalent, not for chronic use
3) Moderate to severe acute or chronic Sx: Pataday 2.5 mL once per day, more frequent dosing may cause irritation
4) For severe Sx, use FML qid with Pataday for a short course

K) Dilating drops
1) Mix 1, 15 mL bottle of 1% Mydriacyl with 1, 5 mL bottle of 10% phenylephrine for quicker drop instillation and better views
2) Must maintain sterile conditions; you are potentially liable if there is a problem
3) Paramyd gives good dilation with less cycloplegia side effect

L) Celluvisc: to cushion a contact fundus or gonio lens, or to lubricate an abrasion

M) 1% Cyclogyl 2, 5, 15 mL: for small abrasions or iritis, lasts 3 – 4 hrs

N) 5% homatropine 5 or 15 mL: for abrasions and foreign bodies, cycloplegia lasts 2 – 4 days

O) 1% atropine 5 or 15 mL: for <u>non-acute</u> iritis, kids with ciliary spasm, cycloplegia lasts 3 – 5 days

P) Glaucoma: see glaucoma chapter for use recommendations
　　1) Once per day beta blockers
　　　　a) Timoptic XE 0.25% and 0.5%, 2.5 and 5 mL
　　　　b) Betagan 0.5%, 2, 5, 10, 15 mL
　　2) Twice per day beta blockers
　　　　a) Timoptic, Betimol 0.25% and 0.5%, 5, 10, 15 mL
　　　　b) Betagan 0.25%, 5 and 10 mL
　　　　c) Betoptic S 0.25%, 2.5, 5, 10, 15 mL
　　　　d) Ocupress 1%, 5 and 10 mL
　　　　e) OptiPranolol 0.3%, 5 and 10 mL
　　3) Other medications
　　　　a) Alphagan P 0.15%, 5, 10, 15 mL
　　　　b) Trusopt 2%, 5 and 10 mL
　　　　c) Xalatan 0.005%, 2.5 mL
　　　　d) Lumigan 0.03%, 2.5 and 5 mL
　　　　e) Travatan Z 0.004%, 2.5 and 5 mL
　　　　f) Azopt 0.5%, 5 mL
　　4) Combinations
　　　　a) Cosopt: 0.5% timolol with Trusopt, 5 and 10 mL
　　　　b) Xalcom: 0.5% timolol with Xalatan
　　　　c) Combigan: 0.5% timolol with Alphagan 0.2%
　　　　d) Extravan: 0.5% timolol with Travatan. Available soon

Notes____

____

____

____

____

____

____

____

2

ORALS FOR EYE CARE

Consult a definitive reference if you lack experience with a drug or if the patient has serious co-morbidity, reduced liver or renal function, or is pregnant or nursing.

A) Convert lbs to kilograms: (lb. - 10%)/2 = kg

B) Antibiotic recommendations: listed in order of preference. See notes and warnings below

1) Lid problems
- Ocular rosacea
- Meibomian gland dysfunction
- Hordeolum
- Chlamydia
  a) Doxycycline: inexpensive, effective, classic
  b) Zithromax: moderate price, use if tetracycline problems or you want simple dosing for an acute problem
  c) Biaxin: expensive, third choice
  d) Tetracycline and erythromycin, inexpensive but not recommended

2) Acute infections with no fever or systemic Sx
- Preseptal cellulitis
- Dacryocystitis
- Hyperacute conjunctivitis
- Sinusitis
- Ear infections
  a) Keflex: inexpensive, effective
  b) Zithromax: moderate price, use for penicillin allergies
  c) Dicloxacillin: moderate price
  d) Augmentin: expensive, very effective, may cause diarrhea
  e) Ceftin: expensive, good for deep complicated infections with multiple organisms
  f) Penicillin, amoxicillin, ampicillin, Bactrim: inexpensive but less effective

C) Penicillins

    1) Dicloxacillin 250 or 500 mg

        a) Indications: broad-spectrum bacterial infections, especially cellulitis. Little staph resistance

        b) Contraindications: penicillin allergy

        c) Adults: 250 – 500 mg qid 1 hr before or 2 hrs after meals

        d) Children: 12 – 25 mg/kg daily, divided qid

        e) Common side effects: allergy

    2) Amoxicillin 250 or 500 mg

        a) Indications: non-serious broad-spectrum bacterial infections, especially sinusitis

        b) Contraindications: penicillin allergy, resistant staph

        c) Adults: 250 – 500 mg qid, OK with meals

        d) Children <20 kg: 20 – 40 mg/kg daily, divided qid

        e) Common side effects: allergy, occasional GI upset and hyperactivity

    3) Augmentin 250 or 500 mg (amoxicillin + clavulanic acid): now also in 200 and 400 mg strengths

        a) Indications: serious or resistant broad-spectrum bacterial infections including beta lactamase staph, a more effective drug

        b) Contraindications: penicillin allergy

        c) Adults and children >40 kg: 500 mg bid

        d) Children <40 kg: 20 – 40 mg/kg daily, divided bid

        e) Common side effects: GI upset, diarrhea, allergy, rash

    4) Penicillin VK 250 or 500 mg

        a) Indications: gonorrhea, strep throat

        b) Contraindications: penicillin allergy, organisms other than gonorrhea or strep

        c) Adults: 500 mg qid, OK with food

        d) Children: 15 – 50 mg/kg daily divided qid

        e) Common side effects: allergy

D) Cephalosporins

    1) Cephalexin (Keflex) 1st generation, 250 or 500 mg

        a) Indications: most gram+ bacterial infections, cellulitis

        b) Contraindications: 10% cross reaction with penicillin allergy, colitis

        c) Adults: 250 – 500 mg qid, OK with food

        d) Children: 25 – 50 mg/kg daily, divided qid

        e) Common side effects: allergy, rash, polyarthritis, diarrhea

    2) Cefuroxime (Ceftin) 2nd generation, 125, 250, 500 mg

        a) Indications: deep and complicated infections by multiple organisms such as in sinusitis and ear infections

        b) Contraindications: 10% cross reaction with penicillin allergy

        c) Adults: 250 – 500 mg bid

        d) Children: 250 mg bid with meal

        e) Common side effects: diarrhea, nausea, vomiting

E) Sulfa
1) Bactrim (sulfa 400 mg + trimethoprim 80 mg), Bactrim DS (sulfa 800 mg + trimethoprim 160 mg), suspension (sulfa 200 mg + trimethoprim 40 mg, per 5 mL)
   - a) Indications: bacterial infection, consider if penicillin allergy and erythromycin causes nausea
   - b) Contraindications: many resistant organisms, sulfa allergies
   - c) Adults: 2 Bactrim bid or 1 Bactrim DS bid
   - d) Children: 40 mg/kg of sulfa, divided bid
   - e) Common side effects: Stevens-Johnson syndrome, colitis (rarely peripheral neuritis, depression, convulsions)

F) Macrolides
1) Zithromax 250 or 500 mg tablets, Z-Pack
   - a) Indications: broad-spectrum bacterial infections. Especially good as a back up for infected patients with penicillin allergies and ocular rosacea/meibomianitis patients intolerant of doxycycline. Drug of choice for chlamydia, 1, 1000 mg dose
   - b) Relative contraindications (coordinate with the medical doctor): concurrent use of theophylline, digoxin, warfarin
   - c) Adults: 500 mg qd first day, then 250 mg qd for 4 days, avoiding antacids, 1 hr before or 2 hrs after meals. Lasts 2 weeks in the body
   - d) Children >6 months: 10 mg/kg qd first day, then 5 mg/kg qd for 4 days
   - e) Common side effects: GI upset, abdominal pain, colitis
2) Biaxin 250 or 500 mg tabs
   - a) Indications: broad-spectrum bacterial infections. For more serious infections than Zithromax
   - b) Contraindications: concurrent use of theophylline, digoxin, lovastatin, cyclosporine, Norpace
   - c) Adults: 250 or 500 mg bid
   - d) Children >20 months: 15 mg/kg/day divided bid
   - e) Common side effects: GI upset, headache, taste changes
3) Erythromycin 250, 333, 500 mg
   - a) Indications: chlamydia in young and child-bearing women, broad-spectrum infection and rosacea/meibomianitis. Inexpensive alternate drug for penicillin allergy patients and doxycycline intolerant patients
   - b) Relative contraindications (coordinate with medical doctor): concurrent use of theophylline, digoxin, cyclosporine, Norpace, prednisone
   - c) Adults: 1000 mg/day divided bid, tid, or qid, OK with meals
   - d) Children: 30 – 50 mg/kg daily divided qid
   - e) Common side effects: nausea is common

G) Tetracyclines
1) Doxycycline 50, 75, 100 mg

       a) Indications: use in place of tetracycline for chlamydia, acne rosacea, meibomian gland disease, good broad-spectrum coverage for infections, good for penicillin allergic patients

       b) Contraindications: children <age 8, and child-bearing women. Will discolor growing teeth. Avoid with concurrent anticoagulants

       c) Adults or >100 lbs: 100 mg bid, avoid milk

       d) Children >age 8: day 1, 2 mg/kg divided bid, then 1 mg/kg qd subsequent days

       e) Common side effects: GI problems, pseudotumor, rashes, *Candida* vaginitis overgrowth, nail discoloration, anemia, dizziness, headache, loss of oral contraceptive effectiveness, photosensitivity (cover skin, wear sunglasses)

H) Antivirals

   1) Acyclovir (Zovirax) 200 mg

       a) Indications: for inexpensive treatment of herpes zoster and herpes simplex infection

       b) Contraindications: difficulty with 5x dosing

       c) Adults with herpes simplex: initially 200 mg 5x/day for 10 days, then 400 mg bid for up to 12 months

       d) Adults with herpes zoster: 800 mg 5x/day for 10 days

       e) Children >2 yrs: 20 mg/kg 5x/day up to 800 mg total per day

       f) Common side effects: headache, CNS changes in elderly, GI upset, vertigo, fatigue

   2) Valtrex 500 mg caps (pro drug of acyclovir)

       a) Indications: more convenient treatment of herpes zoster and herpes simplex infection

       b) Contraindications: cost, concurrent use of probenecid (gout Tx), cimetidine (Tagamet)

       c) Adults with herpes simplex: 1000 mg bid for 10 days, then 500 mg bid for acute ocular herpes. 500 mg bid for suppression of recurrences

       d) Adults with herpes zoster: 1000 mg tid for 7 days

       e) Children: not recommended

       f) Common side effects: GI upset, headache, dizziness

   3) Famvir 125, 250, 500 mg tabs

       a) Indications: more convenient treatment of herpes simplex and herpes zoster infections

       b) Contraindications: cost

       c) Adults with herpes simplex: 125 mg bid until cleared

       d) Adults with herpes zoster: 500 mg tid for 7 days

       e) Children: not recommended

       f) Common side effects: GI upset, insomnia, dizziness, nervousness, fatigue

I) Antihistamines

   1) Loratadine (Claritin) 10 mg: now over-the-counter (OTC)

a) Indications: non-sedating antihistamine for the relief of seasonal allergic Sx. Onset within 1 hr, lasts 24 hrs
b) Contraindications: non-specific
c) Adults and >age 6: 1, 10 mg tab 1 hr before or 2 hrs after meal qd
d) Children <age 6: not recommended
e) Common side effects: GI upset, mucosal dryness, blur, headache, fatigue, sleepiness, hyperkinesia

2) Loratadine + pseudoephedrine sulfate Claritin-D 24 hr 10/240 mg and Claritin-D 12 hr 5/120 mg)
   a) Indications: non-sedating antihistamine and decongestant for the relief of seasonal allergic Sx. If decongestant causes insomnia, use 12 hr version in a.m. and Benadryl in p.m. to aid sleep
   b) Relative contraindications: hypertension, diabetes, ischemic heart disease, narrow angle glaucoma, hyperthyroidism, seizures
   c) Adults and >age 6: 1 tab, 1 hr before or 2 hrs after meal. Once per day for the 24 hr version and bid for the 12 hr version
   d) Children <age 6: not recommended
   e) Common side effects: GI upset, mucosal dryness, blur, headache, fatigue, insomnia, sleepiness, hyperkinesia, appetite suppression, bronchospasm

3) Cetirizine hydrochloride (Zyrtec) 5 or 10 mg tablets and syrup
   a) Indications: non-sedating antihistamine for the relief of allergic Sx
   b) Contraindications: pregnancy, nursing mothers, renal failure
   c) Adults: 10 mg qd
   d) Children 6 – 11 yrs: 5 –10 mg qd
   e) Children 2 – 5 yrs: ½ – 1 teaspoon per day
   f) Common side effects: sleepiness, fatigue, dry mouth

4) Cetirizine hydrochloride 5 mg and pseudoephrine hydrochloride 120 mg (Zyrtec-D 12 hour)
   a) Indications: relief of allergic Sx with nasal congestion
   b) Contraindications: narrow angle glaucoma, hypertension, use of MAO inhibitors (obsolete antidepressant) within 14 days
   c) Adults: 1 tablet bid
   d) Children <12: not recommended
   e) Common side effects: sleepiness, fatigue, dry mouth

5) Diphenhydramine (Benadryl) caps 25 mg OTC
   a) Indications: inexpensive relief of allergic Sx, especially acute and medication induced Sx, sedating
   b) Contraindications: respiratory problems, narrow angle glaucoma, hyperthyroidism, hypertension, cardiovascular disease, GI or urinary obstruction
   c) Adults: 25 – 50 mg qid
   d) Children >6: 25 mg qid
   e) Common side effects: sedation, dizziness, excitement, hypotension, GI upset

6) Diphenhydramine + pseudoephedrine (Benadryl allergy/congestion) caps 25 mg OTC
   a) Indications: inexpensive relief of allergic Sx with nasal congestion
   b) Contraindications: respiratory problems, narrow angle glaucoma, hyperthyroidism, hypertension, cardiovascular disease, GI or urinary obstruction within 2 weeks of MAO inhibitors (obsolete antidepressant)
   c) Adults: 2 caps qid
   d) Children >6: 1 cap qid
   e) Common side effects: sedation, dizziness, excitement, hypotension, rash, GI upset, palpitations

J) Carbonic anhydrase inhibitors: (topical Trusopt is usually a better choice)
  1) Methazolamide (Neptazane) 25 or 50 mg, 100 per bottle
   a) Indications: for reduction of IOP. Fewer side effects than Diamox. Consider Trusopt or Azopt instead
   b) Contraindications: sulfa allergy, concurrent steroid or aspirin use
   c) Adults: 50 – 100 mg bid or tid
   d) Children: not recommended
   e) Common side effects: "tingling" of extremities, tinnitus, fatigue, taste change, GI upset
  2) Acetazolamide (Diamox) 125 or 250 mg tabs, or 500 mg Diamox Sequels
   a) Indications: for IOP reduction. Consider Trusopt or Azopt instead
   b) Contraindications: sulfa allergy, chronic obstructive pulmonary disease, diabetes
   c) Adults, chronic use: Diamox tablets 125 – 250 mg qid or Diamox Sequels 500 mg bid. In angle closure start with a 500 mg loading dose of Diamox (not Sequels)
   d) Children: not recommended
   e) Common side effects: drowsiness, fever, diuresis, malaise, paresthesias, tinnitus, GI distress, blood dyscrasias; half of Diamox patients drop out due to side effects. Diamox Sequels better tolerated

K) Osmotics
  1) Glycerin (Osmoglyn) 50% solution
   a) Indications: urgent relief of angle closure in non-diabetics. Maximum effect in 1 hr. Most effective
   b) Contraindications: diabetes
   c) Adults: 2 – 3 mL/kg of solution, flavored on ice
   d) Children: 2 – 3 mL/kg of solution flavored on ice
   e) Common side effects: nausea, diuresis, vomiting

L) Analgesics & anti-inflammatories

1) Ibuprofen (Advil, Medipren, Midol 200, Motrin, Nuprin) 200 mg per tab
   a) Indications: relief of pain and inflammation
   b) Contraindications: aspirin allergy, alcoholism, gastritis, ulcers, 3rd trimester of pregnancy (use Tylenol instead), concurrent use of other anti-inflammatories such as Celebrex
   c) Adults: 600 – 800 mg tid with food
   d) Children: 10 – 40 mg/kg tid with food
   e) Common side effects: GI upset, dizziness, visual disturbances, photophobia

2) Naproxen (Naprosyn, Naprelan 250 mg, 375 mg, 500 mg) (Aleve 220 mg)
   a) Indications: long acting inflammation and arthritis relief. Less effective than ibuprofen for pain
   b) Contraindications: aspirin allergy, 3rd trimester of pregnancy (see ibuprofen)
   c) Adults: 250 – 500 mg bid, up to 750 mg bid for short term if tolerated
   d) Children: 10 mg/kg divided bid (usually ½ of 250 mg tabs)
   e) Common side effects: GI upset, headache, dizziness, drowsiness, tinnitus, peptic ulcers and bleeding problems, photophobia, heart disease, stroke

3) Tylenol #3 (30 mg codeine + 325 mg acetaminophen)
   a) Indications: inexpensive relief of moderately severe pain
   b) Contraindications: drug abuser, concurrent alcohol use, use of MAO inhibitors (obsolete antidepressant) within 14 days
   c) Adults: 1 – 2 caps every 4 hrs
   d) Children: 0.5 mg/kg of codeine component
   e) Common side effects: sedation, drowsiness, vomiting, constipation, respiratory depression, syncope

4) Celebrex 100 or 200 mg
   a) Indications: arthritis and relief of acute pain. Similar to NSAIDs without stomach problems
   b) Contraindications: sulfa, aspirin, or NSAID allergy
   c) Adults: 200 mg bid with initial loading dose of 400 mg
   d) Children: not recommended <18 yrs
   e) Common side effects: GI upset or pain, blurred vision, increased IOP, cataracts, heart disease, stroke

5) Ultram 50 mg
   a) Indications: relief of moderately severe pain. Non-narcotic but works like narcotics with low risk of addiction. Easy on stomach
   b) Contraindications: opioid allergy, intoxication
   c) Adults 16 – 75 yrs: 50 – 100 mg every 4 – 6 hrs unless liver disease: consider ½ of 50 mg tab for small women and elderly
   d) Children: not recommended

    e) Common side effects: dizziness, nausea, constipation, headache, somnolence, vomiting

6) Vicodin (5 mg hydrocodone bitartrate and 500 mg acetaminophen)
    a) Indications: for relief of moderately severe pain
    b) Contraindications: drug abusers, concurrent alcohol use, use of MAO inhibitors (obsolete antidepressant) within 14 days
    c) Adults: 1 tab every 4 hrs
    d) Children: not approved
    e) Common side effects: depression of respiration and cough reflex, sleepiness

Notes

3

SYSTEMIC MEDICATIONS AND OCULAR SIDE EFFECTS

A) Chloroquine derivatives
1) Chloroquine
a) Old antirheumatic drug
b) Still used for malaria
c) Cause depigmentation of macular retinal pigment epithelium (RPE) and bull's eye maculopathy
d) Retinal damage usually appears after 100 grams cumulative dose
e) Monitor closely with baseline photos, frequent dilated exams, Amsler monocular color vision and macular vision field testing
f) Meds for troops in Persian Gulf, Afghanistan
2) Hydroxychloroquine (Plaquenil)
a) Replaced chloroquine for arthritis treatment
b) Less toxic
c) Antirheumatic
d) 400 mg/day is standard dose
e) Less than 750 mg/day is unlikely to cause chloroquine retinopathy
f) Yearly exams in healthy patients are sufficient (previously, 6 month exams were recommended)

B) Antihistamines
1) OTC: Benadryl and various brands
a) Dryness of mucosal membranes, including eyes
b) Sedation: combining with decongestants (which are stimulants and labeled with -D), minimize drowsiness
c) Dilation of pupils and loss of accommodation in borderline presbyopes is possible
2) Non-sedating (Allegra, Claritin, Zyrtec, Clarinex)
a) Dryness of mucosal membranes
b) Rarely: sedation is possible
c) Dilation and loss of accommodation is possible

C) Phenothiazines and promethazine: Compazine, Phenergan, Thorazine
- 1) Several uses
  - a) Antiemetics
  - b) Antipsychotics
  - c) Antihiccup
  - d) Antitussive
- 2) Anticholinergic side effects: including dryness, sedation, pupil dilation and reduced accommodation
- 3) Rare adverse side effect (temporary): severe eye movement disorders

D) Cardiovascular drugs
- 1) Diuretics: all can cause transient blur due to fluid loss
  - a) Thiazides (Diuril, Hydrochlorothiazide)
    - 1) Sulfa drugs: beware of sulfa allergies
    - 2) Cause potassium depletion
  - b) Loop diuretics (Lasix, Bumex, Demadex)
    - 1) Not sulfa, but cross-react with sulfa allergies [except ethacrynic acid (Edecrin)]
    - 2) Cause potassium depletion
  - c) Potassium sparing diuretics (Diazide, Aldactone, Midamer, Moduretic): combinations with hydrochlorothiazide
  - d) Carbonic anhydrase inhibitors: acetazolamide (Diamox), methazolamide (Neptazane)
    - 1) Sulfa drugs: beware of sulfa allergies
    - 2) Common side effects: kidney stones, loss of appetite, paresthesia, fatigue, headache, bone marrow depression
    - 3) Cause decreased aqueous production in glaucoma
    - 4) Cause decreased cerebral spinal fluid in pseudotumor cerebri
    - 5) Avoid Neptazane in reduced liver function
- 2) Cardiac glycosides: digitalis, digoxin (Lanoxin)
  - a) Used for congestive heart failure, atrial fibrillation, atrial flutter, supraventricular tachycardia
  - b) Very low therapeutic index, easy to overdose and kill
  - c) First signs of overdose
    - 1) Visual disturbances, including hallucinations and color vision changes
    - 2) Nausea
    - 3) Diarrhea
- 3) Antianginals: nitrates
  - a) Any nitrate combined with Viagra, Levitra or Cialis is additive; can cause heart stoppage
    - 1) Short acting sublingual pills: (Nitrostat, Nitrolingual)
    - 2) Long acting pills: (Imdur, Ismo, Dilatrate SR, Isordil)
    - 3) Patches: (Minitran, Nitrodisk, Nitro-Dur)
    - 4) Can cause syncope and color vision disturbances due to vasodilation effects

4) Antiarrhythmics
- a) Local anesthetics or membrane stabilizers: quinidine (Lidocaine, Rythmol, Propafenone)
  - 1) Can produce reversible central vision loss
  - 2) Can produce cognitive impairment
- b) Beta blockers: see examples below in section 5
  - 1) Will negate effectiveness of topical beta blocker
- c) Repolarization prolongation: amiodarone (Cordarone)
  - 1) Cause corneal verticillata (linear pigment streaks in corneal epithelium)
  - 2) Can cause pseudotumor cerebri or optic neuritis
  - 3) Rarely cause sudden permanent retinal damage
  - 4) Can cause pulmonary fibrosis
- d) Calcium channel blockers
  - 1) Examples
    - a) Diltiazem (Cardizem, Dilacor, Tiazac)
    - b) Amlodipine (Norvasc, Lotrel)
    - c) Felodipine (Plendil, Lexxel)
    - d) Isradipine (Dynacirc)
    - e) Nicardipine (Cardene)
    - f) Nifedipine (Adalat, Procardia)
    - g) Nisoldipine (Sular)
    - h) Verapamil (Calan, Isoptin, Verelan, Tarka)
  - 2) Indications
    - a) Arrhythmia
    - b) Angina
    - c) Hypertension
    - d) Migraines
    - e) Raynaud's syndrome
    - f) Congestive heart failure
    - g) May improve optic nerve perfusion in glaucoma
  - 3) Mechanism: vasodilatation of coronary and peripheral vasculature
  - 4) Common side effects: make beta blockers' side effects worse, make the antiplatelet (bleeding) side effect of aspirin worse, possible atrial-ventricular block, possible severe hypotension

5) Beta adrenergic blockers
- a) Examples
  - 1) Acebutolol (Sectral)
  - 2) Atenolol (Tenormin, Tenoretic)
  - 3) Betaxolol (Kerlone)
  - 4) Carteolol: less effect on heart
  - 5) Metoprolol (Toprol, Lopressor)
  - 6) Nadolol (Corgard)
  - 7) Propranolol (Inderal)
  - 8) Timolol (Blocadren)
  - 9) Carvedilol (Coreg)
- b) Indications

       1) Angina
       2) Anxiety
       3) Arrhythmia
       4) Hypertension
       5) Migraine
       6) Myocardial infarction
       7) Supraventricular and sinus tachycardia
   c) Mechanism
       1) Block beta 1 receptors in the heart; slows it
       2) Block beta 2 receptors in lungs and eyes; constrict bronchioles and reduce aqueous production
       3) Dilate blood vessels
   d) Common side effects: bradycardia, asthma exacerbation, fatigue, depression, IOP reduction, will minimize any further IOP reduction from topical beta blockers
6) Angiotensin converting enzyme (ACE) inhibitors
   a) Examples
       1) Benazepril (Lotensin)
       2) Captopril (Capoten)
       3) Enalapril (Vasotec)
       4) Fosinopril (Monopril)
       5) Lisinopril (Prinivil, Zestril)
       6) Quinapril (Accupril)
       7) Ramipril (Altace)
   b) Indications: hypertension, congestive heart failure
   c) Mechanism: intercept the body's natural vasoconstriction mechanism to reduce blood pressure (BP)
   d) Common side effects: rarely blurred vision, cough
7) Angiotensin receptor blockers (ARB)
   a) Example: valsartan (Diovan)
   b) Indications: hypertension, congestive heart failure; fewer side effects than ACE inhibitors
   c) Mechanism: block the body's vasoconstriction mechanism to reduce BP
   d) Common side effects: vertigo, blurred vision
8) Blood thinners
   a) Examples
       1) Aspirin (Bayer, Bufferin, Ecotrin, Plavix)
       2) Heparin (Lovenox)
       3) Warfarin (Coumadin)
   b) Indications
       1) Improve circulation
       2) Decrease clotting
   c) Mechanisms vary
   d) Common side effects: hemorrhage, including ocular. Contraindicated with active intraocular bleeding
9) Cholesterol lowering agents
   a) Bile acid sequestrants
       1) Niacin in megadoses (Niaspan, Nicolar)

           a) Indications: hyperlipidemia
           b) Mechanism: slow bile reabsorption, cholesterol is used to replace bile
           c) Common side effects: flushing (aspirin helps), hypotension, toxic amblyopia, GI upset
        2) Cholestyramine resin (Questran Light)
           a) Indications: hyperlipidemia
           b) Mechanism: slows bile reabsorption, cholesterol is used to replace bile
           c) Common side effects: GI disturbances, vitamin deficiencies could affect vision as well as other health problems
      b) Cholesterol synthesis inhibitors
        1) Examples
           a) Lovastatin (Mevacor)
           b) Pravastatin (Pravachol)
           c) Simvastatin (Zocor)
           d) Atorvastatin (Lipitor)
           e) Rosuvastatin (Crestor)
           f) Ezetimibe/simvastatin combination (Vytorin)
        2) Indications: hyperlipidemia
        3) Mechanism: inhibition of cholesterol synthesis in the liver
        4) Common side effects: early reports of cataract stimulation are not true; rarely conjunctivitis, tearing, blurred vision

E) Isoniazid

    1) Used as part of combination antituberculosis drugs
      a) Examples
        1) Rifamate
        2) Rifater
      b) Common side effects: hepatitis, can cause optic neuropathy

F) Aredia

    1) Used to treat osteoporosis and bone cancer
    2) Reported 17% incidence of scleritis within 2 days of starting medication
    3) Also ocular pain, conjunctivitis, uveitis, episcleritis
    4) Scleritis requires stopping Aredia; the other conditions can be managed
    5) Monitor every 6 months

G) Accutane

    1) Used for severe acne
    2) Usually causes dry eye
    3) Watch for pseudotumor, visual disturbances, decreased night vision, photophobia
    4) Contact lenses contraindicated

H) Tamoxifen
　　1) Used to prevent the recurrence of breast cancer and preventively in high-risk women
　　2) Causes drusen-like deposits in the macula in 1 – 6% of users within 6 months. May also cause keratopathy and optic neuritis
　　3) VA loss is reversible if tamoxifen is discontinued before vision drops below 20/70. Retinal changes are permanent
　　4) Monitor carefully

I) Flomax
　　1) Used to increase urine flow in BPH (benign prostatic hypertrophy) in men and urinary retention in women
　　2) Causes floppy iris syndrome and poor dilation, both of which make cataract surgery more difficult
　　3) The changes appear to be permanent, and discontinuing the drug before surgery does not help

Notes

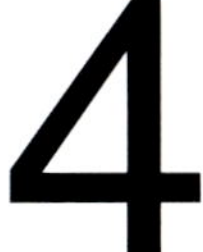

INJURIES

A) Metallic foreign bodies
1) Subjective
   a) Complaints of pain or a foreign body sensation
   b) Ask about a high speed projectile history because penetration can be occult and self-sealing
   c) Ask if occurred at work and if patient was wearing safety glasses because of possible Worker's Compensation insurance questions
   d) Ask about tetanus shot history. If the wound was dirty and bloody and the last booster >10 yrs ago, or did not receive all of boosters, refer for booster shot
2) Objective
   a) VA and pinhole or best corrected VA
   b) Pupils
   c) External
   d) Slit lamp
      1) Instill topical anesthetic if necessary in both eyes to facilitate examination
      2) Look carefully for penetration, dilate if necessary to look for lens penetration and to look at the retina (no scleral depression)
3) Assessment
   a) You must R/O the need for a computerized tomography (CT) or x-ray (no magnetic resonance imaging (MRI))
4) Plan
   a) For limbal or deep conjunctival foreign bodies, soaking a pledget in topical anesthetic and 2.5% phenylephrine and holding on the affected tissue for 1 min will give deeper anesthesia (cocaine in 4% solution or lidocaine 4% are more effective for painful limbal foreign bodies)
   b) Use a foreign body spud, a 1 mm chalazion curette, to remove the foreign body
   c) When using a burr to remove a deep rust ring, rinse and clean the bit frequently
   d) Remove all rust except the lightest staining
   e) Remove all necrotic and edematous material

f) For stromal wounds, instill 5% homatropine. It relieves ciliary spasm for 2 – 3 days, about as long as it takes to heal

g) Instill Acular or Voltaren for pain

h) Instill Polysporin or Ciloxan ointment for prophylaxis and lubrication

i) Pressure patching is becoming controversial, but is still a simple way to relieve pain. If you patch in the morning, have the patient remove it before bed. Afternoon patches need to come off by the next morning. Bandage contact lenses are an alternative

j) Except for non-stromal wounds, prescribe (Rx) Polytrim qid after the patch comes off. If you suspect a contaminated wound, Rx Vigamox or Zymar qid

k) Order a CT whenever an intraocular or orbital foreign body cannot be ruled out (not an MRI)

l) Refer all intraocular foreign bodies to a retina specialist immediately

5) Return to clinic (RTC) in 2 days

   a) Subjective: what % of subjective improvement? Should be at least 50%

   b) Objective: visual acuity (VA), pupils, external, slit lamp

   c) Assessment

      1) Epithelial healing

      2) Stromal edema is likely but no infiltrates should be visible

      3) Watch striae, may indicate edema or early ulcer

      4) Anterior chamber (AC) reaction should be rare cell at most

   d) Plan

      1) Continue the antibiotic x5d

      2) RTC as needed (prn) if Sx worsen or foreign body sensation does not resolve in 3 – 5 days (follow until the epithelium heals)

      3) Consider tears prn if a significant foreign body (FB) sensation exists

B) Abrasions, UV burns, welding burns, chemical splashes

1) Subjective

   a) Severe pain or foreign body Sx

   b) Known history: UV and welding burn symptoms appear several hrs after exposure

2) Objective: (if a chemical burn, irrigate as per Plan below before doing anything else)

   a) Instill topical anesthetic for examination comfort

   b) VA and pinhole or best corrected VA

   c) External

   d) Slit lamp with fluorescein

3) Assessment

   a) Alkali burns (fertilizer, household bleach) are more persistent and destructive than acidic burns

   b) Grade the corneal damage and draw it

    4) Plan
        a) For chemical splashes, always be sure the patient has 30 min of effective irrigation including that done before patient comes to the office. Be sure the lids are held open, or use a speculum
        b) Consider a roll of pH paper. Stop irrigating for 5 min before use. Repeat irrigation until the pH is 7.0
        c) 5% homatropine bid for comfort
        d) Acular or Voltaren qid for comfort
        e) Bacitracin ointment (ung) tid
        f) Pressure patch as needed between ung instillation
        g) Alkali burns with epithelial defects may need up to 1 week of steroid to minimize scarring. Refer if severe or central
    5) RTC in 2 days
        a) Subjective: at least 50% better
        b) Objective
            1) Re-epithelizing
            2) Symblepharon/conjunctival scarring possible with chemical burns
            3) Stromal haze possible
            4) AC reaction possible
        c) Assessment
            1) If central scarring, refer or treat with a steroid
            2) If AC reaction, cycloplegia, consider steroid
        d) Plan: monitor and treat as above until healed
            1) Use bacitracin liberally to lubricate and facilitate healing
            2) If only stromal haze, monitor
            3) If stromal scarring exists after a chemical burn, consider a referral to a cornea specialist or Rx steroids to control

C) Blunt orbital trauma
    1) Subjective
        a) Known history of blunt trauma
        b) Pain?
        c) Decreased vision?
        d) Diplopia?
        e) Flashes or floaters?
    2) Objective
        a) VA: open lids manually if necessary. Pinhole because the habitual Rx may be wrong now
        b) Pupils: afferent pupillary defect (APD) or anisocoria?
        c) Extraocular eye movements
            1) Any pain on eye movement?
            2) Any restrictions, especially in upgaze?
            3) If there is an upgaze restriction, do forced ductions with a cotton tipped applicator soaked in anesthetic if the globe is intact
                a) No restriction indicates a superior rectus paresis

                         b) Restriction indicates a trapped inferior rectus secondary to a blow out fracture

      d) Confrontation fields

      e) Monocular color vision if optic nerve damage suspected

      f) External

            1) Draw and document hemorrhage, ecchymosis, and edema. Many of these cases end up in court and drawings are more useful to lay people on juries

            2) Look for ptosis and lid lacerations

            3) Palpate the orbital rim for step-off fractures and lids for crepitus (crackling sound from trapped air)

            4) Check for hypesthesia of the cheek and upper lip on the affected side compared to the unaffected side

            5) Compare retropulsion of globes (push gently with thumbs) if you do not suspect a ruptured globe

      g) Hertel exophthalmometry: should be ≤ 21 mm and equal

            1) A receded globe may indicate a blow out fracture

            2) A proptotic globe resistant to retropulsion may indicate a retrobulbar hemorrhage

      h) Slit lamp

            1) Cornea: abrasions, lacerations, or striae?

            2) AC: hyphema, free red blood cells, inflammatory cell, pigment or flare?

            3) Iris: any irregular pupil, anisocoria, iris hemorrhage, iridodialysis, sphincter tears or traumatic mydriasis? Compare angle depth between eyes to find angle recession

            4) Lens: subluxation or traumatic cataract? (cataract may take weeks to form)

            5) Pigment or RBC in anterior vitreous

      i) IOP: May be low in a traumatized eye. If very low, consider globe rupture. If high, treat with topical glaucoma meds

      j) Dilated fundus examination (DFE)

            1) Disk pallor or hemorrhage? (pallor may take weeks to form in optic nerve damage)

            2) Retinal hemorrhage or edema from bruising

            3) Macular holes, choroidal rupture, or commotio retinae?

            4) Vitreous hemorrhage or detachment?

            5) Peripheral holes or tears? Do scleral indentation if feasible and no globe penetration or hyphema is present

      k) Gonioscopy: defer for 2 weeks if RBC are present in the AC

    3) Assessment

      a) Identify the affected tissues

      b) If there is decreased vision or color vision without corresponding visible tissue damage, consider traumatic optic neuropathy

      c) If a retinal detachment cannot be ruled out due to a hyphema or vitreous hemorrhage, a B-scan ultrasound should be performed

4) Plan and follow up
    a) Traumatic iritis: 1% cyclopentolate qid or 5% homatropine bid and Pred Forte qid, RTC in 2 days
    b) Hyphema and micro hyphema
        1) Strict bed rest with head elevated 30°
        2) No aspirin or blood thinners
        3) Atropine 1% qid
        4) Pred Forte qid
        5) No reading (too many saccadic eye movements)
        6) TV is good
        7) Treat elevated IOP if necessary
        8) Use a shield on the affected eye
        9) Consider bilateral patching to stop saccades
        10) No strenuous activity or lifting for 2 – 4 weeks
        11) Monitor vision at home and RTC in 1 – 2 days
            a) Monitor fundus as it becomes visible
            b) Do gonioscopy and scleral depression 2 – 4 weeks later
    c) Commotio retinae: monitor weekly, repeat scleral depression
    d) Choroidal rupture: retinal consult, then monitor weekly, then monthly for neovascular membrane formation
    e) Orbital blow out, superior rectus paresis, crepitus, rim fracture, hypesthesia, exophthalmos resistant to retropulsion
        1) Instruct not to blow nose
        2) Immediately (STAT) CT
        3) Referral to oculoplastics ophthalmologist, or ENT if CT is positive
        4) Start broad-spectrum antibiotics and a nasal decongestant
    f) Traumatic optic neuropathy: STAT referral for CT and possible steroids and optic nerve sheath fenestration
    g) Laceration, penetration, or rupture of globe or cornea: STAT referral to appropriate sub specialist, usually retina or cornea, depending on location of injury

Notes

5

RED EYE MISCELLANEOUS

A) Lids and margins
1) Subjective: from no Sx to itching and burning lids to intense pain
2) Objective
   a) Blepharitis: flakes to heavy crusting with lid redness and swelling, foam along lid margin
   b) Meibomian gland disease (MGD)
      1) Telangiectasia: look carefully at lid margins and note facial rosacea
      2) Express meibomians on all 4 lids. Note capping
   c) Hordeolum (stye) or chalazion: note and draw size and location
3) Assessment
   a) Blepharitis: grade for reference as you follow improvement
   b) MGD grading scale
      1) Grade 0: light, clear, oily secretion easily expressed
      2) Grade 1: "milky" secretion easily expressed
      3) Grade 2: "chunky, greasy" secretions are expressed, also see chunks floating in tear film after expression
      4) Grade 3: "toothpaste" squeeze expressed with resistance
      5) Grade 4: "toothpaste" squeeze expressed with high resistance or not at all (use 2 opposing cotton tipped applicators)
   c) Hordeolum: note if it is erupting or pointing
   d) Chalazion: long standing, non-painful, not red, lump. R/O skin cancer
4) Plan
   a) Blepharitis: soak and scrub bid OU
      1) Very warm compresses every 5 – 10 min
      2) Thorough scrubbing of lid margins with lid scrub soap, preferably anti-bacterial
      3) Rinse
      4) Severe cases will benefit from bacitracin ung bid on margins
      5) If marked lid margin inflammation, use Tobradex ung
      6) RTC in 2 weeks
   b) MGD

1) Soak and scrub tid if possible. Hot soaks are even more important
2) Squeeze out the meibomian glands in a milking action
3) Topicals are little help
4) In severe cases, Rx doxycycline 100 mg bid po (unless pregnant or growing child) until improves and then 50 – 100 mg qd for long term maintenance
5) RTC in 2 weeks
  c) Hordeolum
1) Cannot excise until it quiets
2) For lots of heat delivery, boil an egg or microwave a potato and wrap in a damp washcloth and apply to the lid
3) If painful, Rx doxycycline with heat
4) If pointing: express, open if necessary (only if pointing!)
5) RTC in 2 – 4 days
  d) Chalazion
1) Inject 0.2 – 1 mL of Kenalog unless darkly pigmented (this may depigment the skin)
2) Excision is the most common procedure. If recurrent, send to pathology to R/O cancer
3) RTC prn if no procedure done

B) Dry eye

1) Subjective
  a) History of dry, scratchy or foreign body sensation, or transient blur improving with blink
  b) In teen, ask about Accutane use
  c) Possible Sjögren's Sx such as dry mouth
  d) Sx may wax and wane according to environmental conditions such as humidity, air conditioning, etc.
  e) 8% of women >age 50 affected
2) Objective
  a) May have blepharitis or meibomianitis which may be contributing to a dry eye, or the entire cause for Sx
  b) Corneal and/or conjunctival staining with fluorescein
  c) Minimal tear prism
  d) Poor tear quality or break up time <5 sec
3) Assessment
  a) R/O lid disease
  b) R/O epithelial basement membrane disease (EBMD), foreign bodies, and other corneal problems
  c) Determine if it is a tear quality problem (matter or greasy chunks in tears, poor break up time) or a tear volume problem (small tear prism or reduced Schirmer's with anesthetic)
4) Plan
  a) Tear quality problems are usually caused by meibomianitis
1) Mild to moderate: Rx hot soaks and lid scrubs bid or more with tears prn

       2) Severe: oral tear quality treatment for meibomianitis and rosacea. Beware of causing or aggravating cholesterol problems with the oils. Always use non-preserved tears, hot compresses and lid scrubs concurrently
- a) Flaxseed oil 1 gram bid po with meal
- b) Fish oil 1 – 2 grams per day
- c) Doxycycline 100 mg po bid for 1 month then qd for 2 months

   b) Tear volume problems, a staged approach
- 1) Mild: preserved tears 1 – 3x/day
- 2) Moderate: non, or minimally preserved tears such as Genteal, TheraTears, Refresh Liquigel, Systane, Refresh Plus, or Optive, if dosing of 4x or more is needed to prevent confusion with solution sensitivity problems later. Overnight protection with Refresh Plus gel may also be needed
- 3) Advanced
  - a) Punctal plugs with non-preserved lubrication as needed
  - b) Restasis (cyclosporine 0.05%) bid or topical FML qid as inexpensive trial. Expect 1 – 3 month delay in Sx improvement, especially if inflammatory component suspected
- 4) Severe tear volume problem or Sjögren's
  - a) Use topical anti-inflammatory treatment in addition to plugs and lubrication and possibly goggles
  - b) Add oral treatment: Salagen (oral pilocarpine) 5 mg bid to start, then qid. Half fail due to GI upset though

C) Conjunctiva: itchy-scratches/red eye differential

   1) Subjective: history is very important
- a) If history of exposure to someone with a red eye, probably viral etiology and is contagious
- b) Ask if recent upper respiratory infection (URI) symptoms such as sore throat or rhinitis
- c) For subconjunctival hemorrhage ask about lifting, straining, constipation, blood thinners, aspirin, and supplements such as garlic, ginger, ginseng, ginkgo biloba
- d) Ask about itching vs. burning, stinging, scratchiness
- e) Ask if lids are matted shut or have purulent discharge. Is there ropy mucus or slippery tears?

   2) Objective
- a) Palpable or tender pre-auricular nodes (PAN): sometimes helpful, document
- b) Look at margins and meibomians
- c) Grade the amount of, and color of, injection
- d) Grade the chemosis
- e) Note any follicles: rarely helpful but document
- f) Note presence of and quality of mucus
- g) Draw subconjunctival heme

h) R/O iritis and angle closure
i) Always take BP with subconjunctival heme
3) Assessment
    a) Allergic conjunctivitis: itchy, ropy mucus, slippery tears, mild injection, more chemosis, environmental correlation
    b) Viral conjunctivitis: much more common than bacterial, burning, prominent mucus including matting shut is possible, "pink" injection, follicles and PAN may (or may not) be present. History usually indicates contagious exposure and infection starting in one eye followed by the other eye
    c) Bacterial conjunctivitis: bacterial conjunctivitis without blepharitis is actually quite rare and usually over diagnosed. Beefy redness and prominent mucus are common
    d) Subconjunctival hemorrhage: pooling of blood in an asymptomatic eye
4) Plan
    a) Allergic
        1) Mild to moderate: Similasan Allergy Eye Relief
        2) Moderate to severe: Pataday qd – bid may be necessary (note, higher doses may cause burning and dryness)
        3) Severe may need FML or Alrex qid until controlled enough for Patanol
        4) RTC in 1 – 2 weeks
    b) Viral
        1) Counsel about hygiene, frequent hand washing, personal wash cloths, clean pillowcases
        2) Counsel that the patient is likely to be contagious as long as the eye is tearing
        3) Rx vasoconstrictors or tears as needed
        4) FML if serious subjective and objective findings (such as infiltrates in the visual axis)
        5) RTC in 1 week
    c) Bacterial
        1) Treat lids with scrubs even if they look clean; this will reduce the bacteria reservoir around eye where drops are not effective
        2) Rx Polytrim qid – q2h
        3) RTC in 2 – 5 days
    d) Subconjunctival hemorrhages
        1) Do not blow them off!
        2) Take BP!
            a) Systolic >220 or diastolic >115 with end organ damage (subconjunctival heme) is an emergency. If the medical doctor cannot see the patient immediately, send to the emergency department
            b) If hypertensive, do at least direct ophthalmoscopy to check for papilledema or other retinopathy
            c) RTC prn unless eye pathology is found

D) Contact lens associated red eye (CLARE)
    1) Subjective
        a) History of contact lens wear recently or presently, especially soft or overnight wear (even with silicone hydrogel), dirty lenses, non-compliance with lens replacement schedules
        b) Red eye, epiphora
        c) Pain or foreign body sensation
        d) Photophobia
        e) Blur
    2) Objective
        a) VA may be normal or reduced
        b) If the lens is still in, it may be fitting tightly
        c) Conjunctival injection, local, limbal, or diffuse
        d) Mattering possible
        e) Corneal edema, infiltration, staining, and ulceration are all possible
        f) AC cell, flare, or pigmentation are all possible
    3) Assessment
        a) Is there only epithelial edema or stromal striae?
        b) Is there white blood cell infiltration, especially near the limbus?
        c) Is there epithelial staining and cell death?
        d) Is there a frank ulcer with cloudy infiltration of the stroma vs. an anterior stromal reaction on the surface of the stroma?
    4) Plan
        a) For edema only, remove the lenses and use lubrication drops prn for comfort. RTC in 2 days. No lens wear for one month, re-check the fit, re-instruct on wearing schedules if necessary
        b) For infiltration, stop lens wear and Rx Tobradex qid. RTC in 1 day to be sure not progressing to ulceration or HSV
        c) For subepithelial infiltrates with staining, stop lens wear and Rx Vigamox q2h. After re-epithelialization, add Pred Forte qid. Alternatively, Tobradex q2h if there is no suspicion of ulceration. RTC daily until improvement noted
        d) For a true corneal ulcer with white blood cells (WBC) or infiltrates in the stroma, striae, AC reaction, but not large or central
            1) Remove contacts
            2) Rx Vigamox q5 min for 1 hr then q30 min during the day and q1h at night. Alternatively Polysporin ung hs can be used for the nighttime dosing
            3) Rx 5% homatropine bid for pain
            4) RTC in 1 day
        e) Large or central true ulcer
            1) Do Gram stain and culture on blood, chocolate, thioglycolate broth and Sabouraud's or refer to be done. If using culturette, be sure to moisten swab first by breaking vial
            2) Refer for fortified antibiotics. Vigamox and Zymar may be as effective, but are not FDA approved for ulcers yet

E) Cornea
1) Subjective: from scratchy, foreign body sensation to intense pain
2) Objective
   a) Look carefully with a good slit lamp and white light for epithelial erosions, filaments, epithelial basement membrane disease, striae, infiltrates, endothelial loss or keratitic precipitates (KPs), AC reaction
   b) Stain lightly with fluoro-strip and look for the staining pattern. Fluress is too viscous and will hide light staining
3) Assessment
   a) Punctate epithelial erosions (PEE): only see after stain. Mild damage
   b) Punctate epithelial keratitis (PEK): see white defects before stain. May cause positive or negative stain. More damage. This grading system will allow you to more closely follow healing or deterioration
   c) Superficial punctate keratitis (SPK): this term is only correct in Thygeson's disease
   d) Overall pattern: virus, dry eye, eye drop sensitivity
   e) Inferior ⅓ stain line pattern: assume staph marginal keratitis or lagophthalmos
   f) Note if diffuse or confluent stain pattern, draw
   g) Do not use too much fluorescein; look carefully for negative stain, indicating an elevated area (epithelial basement membrane disease, HSV keratitis or Thygeson's)
   h) AC reaction up to hypopyon is possible: look at the inferior angle!
   i) Striae
   j) WBC or infiltrate in stroma vs. "anterior stromal reaction"
   k) Is the stain pooling in a depression or is it staining cells (dendrite vs. pseudo-dendrite, staining Lasik flap vs. normal flap gutter)?
      1) Form a fine strand of cotton on a cotton tip applicator
      2) Wick away fluorescein; if pooling, it will disappear, if staining it will stay stained
   l) Deep achy pain and photophobia
   m) Prepare slide for Gram stain, culture on blood, chocolate, thioglycolate broth and Sabouraud's. Use sterile spatula or spud
4) Plan
   a) Filaments
      1) Remove by rotating a sterile cotton tipped applicator moistened with anesthetic
      2) Rx topical antibiotics and aggressive non-preserved tear application
      3) Avoid ointments
      4) Consider temporary disposable CL with antibiotic use; it will melt filaments beneath the lens
      5) Treat the cause of the filaments

      6) RTC in 2 days
   b) Subepithelial infiltrates: epidemic keratoconjunctivitis
      1) Lubricate and counsel if few Sx
      2) Probably not infectious at this stage, but wash your hands anyway!
      3) Instill topical anesthetic
      4) Instill 1 drop of ophthalmic Betadine
      5) Irrigate well
      6) Rx FML or Tobradex qtt qid
      7) RTC in 2 – 4 days
   c) Bacterial keratitis
      1) Simple bacterial keratitis
         a) Polytrim qid – q2h
         b) Lid hygiene
         c) RTC in 2 days unless CL related, pain increases or vision decreases
      2) Staph marginal infiltrates without AC reaction
         a) Tobradex q2h or Vigamox qid with Pred Forte qid
         b) Lid hygiene
         c) RTC in 2 days unless CL related, pain increases, or vision decreases
      3) True corneal ulcers or CL related
         a) Start on Vigamox q5 min for 1 hr then q30 min during day and q1h at night if bad. Polysporin ung hs if less worrisome. Tobradex ung hs can be used later if need steroid for scarring
         b) Rx 5% homatropine bid for pain
         c) RTC in 1 day
         d) Pred Forte qid after ulcer is healing and sterile
      4) Large or central true corneal ulcer
         a) Refer or do stain and culture, and then refer for fortified antibiotics
         b) Vigamox and Zymar may be as effective as fortified antibiotics without the toxicity for most pathogens, but they are not FDA approved for ulcers yet
      5) Fungal ulcer
         a) History (Hx) of vegetative abrasion or a chronically sick eye
         b) Gray feathery infiltrate, satellite lesions
         c) Very painful, little pus
         d) Does not respond to antibiotics
         e) REFER!
      6) Acanthamoeba
         a) Ring stromal infiltrate around the ulcer
         b) Usually a CL wearer or a swimming Hx
         c) Unusually painful!
         d) Non-responsive to antibiotics
         e) REFER!

      d) EBMD
          1) If the epithelium is loosely attached
              a) Debride it back to healthy margins with a spud, forceps
              b) Lightly abrade Bowman's membrane with an Alger
                  brush to facilitate epithelial attachment
          2) Instill cyclopentolate or 5% homatropine for ciliary spasm
          3) Instill Voltaren for comfort
          4) Instill bacitracin ung and pressure patch for up to 24 hrs,
             then Rx bacitracin ung tid
          5) Alternatively, insert a bandage lens and Rx Polytrim gtt qid
          6) RTC in 2 days
          7) Use 5% NaCl ung hs for 2 months
          8) If recurrent, try stromal micropuncture
          9) If still recurrent, consider excimer PTK

F) Herpes simplex virus (HSV)
    1) Subjective: usually unilateral, red, photophobic, tearing
    2) Objective
        a) May have lid or skin involvement
        b) May have tender or palpable pre auricular nodes
        c) Look for dendrites with end bulbs
        d) Compare corneal sensitivities with cotton wisp
        e) Look for cells and flare
        f) Measure IOP
    3) Assessment: R/O pseudo-dendrite (a healing abrasion line) by
        a) History: ask how it felt yesterday. If it was a lot worse, it is a
            healing abrasion. If pain is worse today, it is a likely HSV
            dendrite
        b) Pseudo-dendrites do not have end bulbs that stain with rose
            bengal or lissamine green
        c) If you are still unsure of diagnosis, lubricate with bacitracin
            ung and RTC in 1 day. If worse, treat as HSV
    4) Plan
        a) Be sure patient is off of any steroid
        b) Consider gentle debridement of dendrite with sterile cotton
            tipped applicator to reduce viral load (experts disagree)
        c) Rx Viroptic 1% 9x/day (q1h – q2h)
        d) Pediatric use: if the child is uncooperative with drops and
            tearing is diluting the Viroptic, co-manage with pediatrician to
            Rx acyclovir, Valtrex, or Famvir. 2 or more yrs of slow taper
            may be necessary
        e) Instill 5% homatropine (or atropine 1% if severe)
        f) RTC in 2 days, draw and monitor ulcer size
        g) Viroptic 5 – 9x/day for 2 weeks then taper for 1 week, lubricate
            with bacitracin ung
        h) If there is still a remaining defect, need to discontinue Viroptic
            because it becomes toxic and it may be the reason for the
            defect. If no rose bengal stain, probably no active virus; lube
            aggressively and watch

       i) If you need further viral coverage, Rx oral acyclovir 200 mg po 5x/day or Valtrex 500 mg po bid, or Famvir 125 mg po bid. Consult with an internist if kidney problems or pregnancy

       j) Stromal reaction under dendrite, watch carefully, should fade gradually

      k) Stromal disease: REFER!

         1) Disciform: disk shaped stromal edema with intact epithelium, local KPs, possible mild iritis

         2) Necrotizing interstitial: multiple or diffuse infiltrates with thinning, neovascularization, inflammation. Possible hypopyon, iritis and glaucoma

         3) Neurotrophic ulcer: a sterile, melting ulcer

G) Herpes zoster (HZO) (shingles)

    1) Subjective: pain, usually intense on one side of the face

    2) Objective

      a) VA and pinhole or best corrected VA

      b) External: note and draw vesicles and note if they are wet or dry

      c) Versions to R/O extra ocular muscles (EOM) palsy

      d) IOP: glaucoma is a common side effect of HZO

      e) Slit lamp: conjunctivitis, diffuse corneal staining, pseudo-dendrites from mucus plaques, and iritis may be present

      f) DFE: important to R/O rare but devastating retinitis or vitritis

    3) Assessment: HZO respects the midline (vs. HSV)

    4) Plan

      a) Treat any IOP rise, iritis or corneal staining in the usual way

      b) Treat IOP without prostaglandins if iritis is present

      c) Be sure the patient is on antivirals or you will need to Rx acyclovir 800 mg 5x/day or Valtrex 1000 mg bid (if not pregnant or renal failure) for 10 days

      d) Tylenol 3 and Zostrix may be needed for skin neuralgia (keep out of the eye), very painful

      e) If the eye is unaffected, RTC in 1 month and repeat exam for late onset ocular complications

H) Episcleritis

    1) Subjective: red eye with painless to moderate pain or tenderness

    2) Objective

      a) Sectorial or diffuse deep injection of episclera. Nodules are possible, often with pingueculae

      b) R/O iritis

    3) Assessment

      a) R/O conjunctivitis by clinical examination. Also 2.5% Neo-Synephrine will blanch conjunctivitis quickly, but not episcleritis

      b) R/O scleritis: scleritis pain is usually deep, severe and radiating. Scleritis causes extreme sensitivity to touch or pressure through the closed lid. Scleritis redness will not blanch with 10% phenylephrine, episcleritis will

4) Plan
- a) Mild: tears prn
- b) Moderate: FML qid
- c) Severe: Pred Forte qid or more, ibuprofen 400 mg po qid
- d) RTC in 1 week
- e) Consider other connective tissue disease

I) Scleritis

1) Subjective: may be deep, severe, radiating pain, red eye, very sensitive to touch through the closed lid
2) Objective
- a) Injection of deep vessels and purple or blue tinge of sclera observed with normal room lighting
- b) Nodules may be present
3) Assessment
- a) Vessels are not mobile with cotton swab
- b) Vessels do not blanch with 10% phenylephrine
- c) Pain is usually intense
- d) Iritis, corneal, lens, retinal changes may co-exist; do a dilated fundus exam
- e) Many have connective tissue disease
4) Plan
- a) Internal medicine or rheumatology consult
- b) Oral prednisone 80 mg po in divided doses until improvement, then slow taper
- c) Ibuprofen 600 mg qid po
- d) RTC in 2 days
- e) Refer if no improvement in 1 week

Notes____

____

____

____

____

____

____

____

____

____

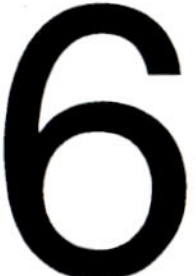

6

DIAGNOSIS AND MANAGEMENT OF UVEITIS

A) Subjective: diagnose by the classic history
1) Acute iritis or uveitis causes a red painful photophobic eye
2) Ask, "Is it an itchy scratchy pain (cornea or external disease), or deep and achy (uveitis)?"
3) Acute uveitis pain is invariably deep and achy, usually intense and debilitating
4) The affected eye has a photophobic reaction when light is shone in the contralateral eye
5) Chronic smoldering uveitis may have no pain and a white eye
6) Juvenile uveitis is more likely to be severe and chronic

B) Objective
1) VA (corrected) and pinhole VA if necessary (grade II+ − IV+ cells may cause complaints of hazy vision)
2) Pupils: may be miotic from ciliary spasm. R/O APD
3) External: blepharospasm and deep conjunctival injection (red-purple color) and ciliary flush. Look for herpes simplex or zoster vesicles. Look for subtle sarcoid nodules in the lid margin and on the conjunctiva
4) Slit lamp: use a good slit lamp
   a) Cornea
      1) Epithelium: use stain to R/O any HSV dendrite or bacterial ulcer as a precipitating factor. Remember we will be using steroids
      2) Stroma: clear and compact unless other problems
      3) Endothelium: look for KPs
         a) Draw: note
            1) Number
            2) Size
            3) Distribution: (superior KPs usually are herpes simplex)
         b) Type
            1) Granulomatous (mutton fat) KPs
            2) Non-granulomatous
             3) Fine dusting: (too fine to see except in retroillumination)
         c) Age (difficult judgment)

           1) New: appears wet or cheesy
           2) Old: dry, dusty, pigmented, involuted
      b) AC reaction: qualify and quantify
         1) Look for cell and flare before using any drops
         2) Use brightest parallelepiped about the size of the pupil to find cell and flare. Back-scattered light from the iris will wash out view if the beam is too large
         3) Look in front of black pupil, but search the entire chamber
         4) Grade cell (looks like small white spheres), flare (looks like smoke or white lint), and pigment individually with a 1 mm² spot beam directed from as far to side as possible
         5) Iritis grading system: cell is diagnostic for follow up as the iritis resolves
            a) Rare: 1 or less cell in 1 mm² beam
            b) Occasional: 3 cells in 1 mm² beam
            c) ½+: 5 cells in a 1 mm² beam
            d) I+: 10 cells in a 1 mm² beam
            e) II+: 20 cells in a 1 mm² beam
            f) III+: 30 cells in a 1 mm² beam
            g) IV+: 40 cells in a 1 mm² beam (driving through blizzard with headlights on)
         6) Grade pigment and flare with the same scale
         7) Is the aqueous plasmoid? Do the cells circulate or are they fixed? If plasmoid, the increased fibrin levels indicate a more severe iritis and cause an increased risk of synechiae. A plasmoid aqueous may also indicate ciliary body shut-down
         8) Is there a hypopyon or individual red blood cells? Indicates human leukocyte antigens (HLA)-B27 or possibly Behcet's or an endogenous endophthalmitis
         9) Is the chamber deep, no peripheral anterior synechiae?
      c) Iris
         1) Look for posterior synechiae, but can't tell for sure until dilate
         2) Look for iris nodules (granulomatous)
         3) Look for iris atrophy or color change (Fuch's heterochromic iridocyclitis). Sector atrophy and transillumination defects are probably herpes simplex
      d) Lens
         1) Not diagnostic unless hypermature cataract causing inflammation, trauma, or posterior synechiae
         2) If pseudophakic, R/O UGH (uveitis, glaucoma, hyphema)
   5) IOP
     1) Usually low: OK
     2) If high: treat, avoid prostaglandins. Do not use optipranolol or pilocarpine. Do not do argon laser trabeculoplasty (ALT)
     3) If dangerously high, consider Fuch's or glaucomatocyclitic crisis (Posner-Schlossman)
       a) IOP may be 40 – 60

　　　　　　　b) Mild AC reaction
　　　　　　　c) Mild, fine KPs on cornea or in trabecular meshwork
　　　　　　　d) Start glaucoma meds and topical steroid
　　　6) Dilated fundus examination: cycloplegia causes dramatic relief of pain. If necessary, do this earlier to facilitate other examination
　　　　　a) Check for synechiae: break if present
　　　　　　　1) Tropicamide 1% and 2.5% phenylephrine, wait ½ hr
　　　　　　　2) Try Tropicamide 1% and 10% phenylephrine, wait ½ hr
　　　　　　　3) Soak a pledget with Tropicamide 1% and 10% phenylephrine and insert under lower lid while looking up with topical anesthesia for 5 – 10 min if necessary. Alternatively, use 5 doses of 10% phenylephrine 5 min apart. Punctal occlude and monitor BP and pulse for systemic reaction, especially if cardiac risk factors
　　　　　　　4) Many will break later at home
　　　　　b) Do DFE if feasible, R/O rare but dangerous problems that require a STAT retina consult. If photophobia is too intense, do it at the next visit
　　　　　　　1) Intermediate uveitis: cells in anterior vitreous, unknown origin, may spill over into or from the AC. Consult
　　　　　　　2) Pars planitis: the most missed diagnosis. You must scleral depress at least inferiorly. Look for snowballs/snowbanks especially at inferior equator. Often indicates Lyme disease. Retina consult
　　　　　　　3) Histo or toxo scars: inspect closely for fluffy lesions at the edge of an old scar. Consult (STAT if near macula)
　　　　　　　4) Look for exudation from vessels or disk. STAT consult
　　　　　　　5) Look for cystoid macular edema (CME), especially if VA is down. Retinal inflammation can cause epiretinal membranes after time. Retina consult
　　　　　　　6) Look for an exudative choroiditis or acute retinal necrosis. STAT consult

C) Assessment: these conditions are easier to treat
　　　1) **Subclinical iritis**: mild to moderate classic Sx, but no objective signs
　　　2) **Anterior uveitis** or iritis vs. intermediate uveitis vs. pars planitis vs. pan uveitis
　　　　　a) 95% of uveitis is anterior
　　　　　b) Intermediate uveitis: inflammation affecting the ciliary body, vitreous, and peripheral retina
　　　　　c) Pars planitis is a subset of intermediate uveitis characterized by inflammation at the pars plana
　　　3) **Unilateral** vs. bilateral: bilaterality indicates a systemic cause that will need a laboratory workup. Expect the uveitis to be harder to treat
　　　4) **Initial** or recurrent? (3rd or greater occurrence) 50% of recurrent uveitis has a systemic cause

5) **Idiopathic** (50%) vs. systemic cause

D) Plan
1) Cycloplegia
    a) 1 drop of atropine in office
        1) Use only if a low risk of synechiae such as in traumatic or post surgical iritis
        2) With any other iritis it may get much worse before you get it under control. Avoid synechiae in an 8 mm pupil. They are usually not breakable
        3) Lasts about 1 week: inexpensive
    b) 1 drop of 5% homatropine in office: only if low risk of synechiae, lasts 1 – 3 days
        1) Subclinical iritis
        2) Traumatic iritis
        3) Post-surgical iritis
        4) Staph marginal infiltrates causing ciliary spasm or AC reaction
        5) Post foreign body removal ciliary spasm or AC reaction
    c) Cyclopentolate 1% bid – tid for all other uveitis: preferred, mobility prevents synechiae. Pharmacy may not carry; dose in-office to start
    d) Tropicamide 1% tid also OK
2) Steroid: Pred Forte is preferred. Inflamase Forte has a better, inexpensive generic and patients do not have to remember to shake. Use only Pred Forte for III+ or greater iritis. This is an initial dosing plan. The most common mistake is under-treatment. Dark irides need more steroids
    a) Grade occasional cell, or traumatic, or subclinical iritis: Rx qid
    b) Grade I+ – II+ cell: Rx q2h (waking)
    c) Grade III cell: Rx q1h
    d) Grade IV cell and plasmoid aqueous: q30 min. Consider adding FML or Tobradex ung hs
    e) Granulomatous: consider sending out for a conjunctival biopsy before using steroids
        1) Ocular sarcoidosis affects only the eye, blood tests will not detect unless lung involvement
        2) Later, if the treatment is not working and you are trying to R/O ocular sarcoid, a biopsy will not help because topical steroids will have melted the sarcoid nodules
3) RTC in 2 days, nothing will change sooner for up to grade III cell. RTC in 1 day for grade IV cell or plasmoid aqueous

E) 2 day follow up
1) Subjective: ask how much improvement of symptoms in percentage. Expect about 50% from cycloplegia, even if AC is no better
2) Objective: VA, IOP, slit lamp. Do DFE if not done yet

3) Assessment/Plan: is it improving?
    a) Improving: continue cycloplegia and steroid according to the above guidelines. RTC in 2 days
    b) Unchanged: increase meds 1 step. RTC in 2 days
    c) Worse: repeat DFE, increase to max meds. RTC in 1 day
    d) If still synechiae, repeat pledget, monitor BP

F) Continuing follow up

1) Long term steroid can cause IOP rise (usually after 3 – 8 weeks) and posterior subcapsular cataracts, but there is no alternative here. Watch for side effects and treat as needed
2) If still worsening, still grade IV+, hypopyon, or any posterior chamber involvement: get consult urgently
3) If unchanged (and does not meet criterion in F2) with controllable IOP, do uveitis questionnaire (see end of chapter) and lab testing (section J below). Sit tight for 2 weeks at max topical meds. Then consider consultation and oral prednisone or Kenalog injection
4) If improving
    a) Continue Pred dosing until only rare or occasional cells in AC
    b) Simple, acute iritis that responds quickly: taper with 2 day steps
        1) Example taper steps: q30 min, q1h, q2h, qid, tid, bid, qd
    c) Chronic, recurrent, systemic, slow responding cases need 1 week – 1 month steps
    d) Be prepared to medicate for months in stubborn cases but do not under medicate. Always monitor IOP and watch for CME
    e) A damaged blood aqueous barrier in the ciliary body can leak protein flare permanently. Only treat cell
    f) Long standing trace cell can eventually cause CME
    g) Lotemax can be substituted if necessary for steroid responders after you achieve control. Increase Lotemax dosage 1 level if substituted for Pred Forte. Using the same dosage counts as a taper step because Lotemax is less potent
5) Get a consult if indicated
6) Fuch's heterochromic iridocyclitis etiology may be viral. Steroids are of limited help. Refer
7) Use topical Acular and Pred Forte with Indocin 25 mg tid po (or ibuprofen 600 mg tid po) for CME. Discontinue topical epinephrine, Propine, Xalatan, which can cause CME
8) Bilateral scleritis is a very serious problem: REFER!

G) Kenalog injections: for powerful long term control with few systemic side effects

1) Used for
    a) Any anterior uveitis that cannot be controlled topically
    b) Any posterior uveitis
2) 10 – 40 mg injected sub-tenon superior and/or inferior

3) Lasts about 2 months. You can see the off-white cheesy deposits under the conjunctiva
4) Can also be injected retrobulbar with the same effectiveness. Less discomfort? Most ophthalmologists are more familiar with doing this procedure
5) Monitor IOP for several months; if severe steroid response, the deposit may need to be excised or a trabeculectomy performed. ⅓ have an IOP rise

H) Oral prednisolone: (10 – 60 mg) alternative to Kenalog; do not want to use for a chronic iritis with systemic cause because of systemic side effects
   1) Be sure no diabetes. Monitor glucose weekly
   2) If diabetic, monitor glucose daily and only with an internist's help
   3) Be sure no stomach ulcer Hx
   4) Taper orals first, then topicals

I) Methotrexate and cyclosporine: antimetabolites used for chemotherapy. Low doses are used for chronic uveitis and other connective tissue disorders
   1) Only used by uveitis expert or in conjunction with an experienced internist
   2) Can be very effective in reducing the need for steroid or in getting recalcitrant, chronic cases under control
   3) Good for rheumatoid and juvenile rheumatoid arthritis-related uveitis

J) Laboratory testing for uveitis/iritis: iritis is often a sign and symptom of systemic disease
   1) Consider laboratory investigation when
      a) Third or greater occurrence
      b) Bilateral
      c) Granulomatous (larger, white KPs)
      d) Slow resolving (>6 weeks) or flaring iritis
      e) Significant positive uveitis questionnaire results (see end of chapter)
      f) Posterior or intermediate uveitis (also order a retina/uveitis consult)
   2) Sources of privileges
      a) Local hospital
      b) Local for profit lab
      c) Local friendly medical doctor
   3) Write out requested tests with diagnosis on your Rx pad and send with the patient
   4) If no privileges are possible, phone the patient's medical doctor, give the differential diagnosis and what you need to R/O and the indicated lab tests. Do not insult him/her, but some tests are better for our purposes than others

5) Order lab tests to R/O systemic conditions. Refer to an internist as necessary for systemic treatment. Expect slow resolution and recurrences if a systemic factor identified. Use 1 week – 1 month per step taper
6) A basic limited screen recommended for all uveitis patients
   a) Complete blood count (CBC) with platelet and differential: good overall health screening. Normals are listed on the lab report
      1) A high platelet count with chronic bilateral uveitis indicates a lymphoma
      2) A high white blood cell count indicates a systemic infection
   b) Westergren erythrocyte sedimentation rate (sed rate): non-specific, indicates systemic inflammation, infection, malignancy, or collagen vascular disorder versus local inflammation (*i.e.*, idiopathic uveitis). Maximum normal values for males are age $\div 2$. For females (age $+10$)$\div 2$
   c) Fluorescent treponemal antibody absorption (FTA-ABS): best syphilis test. You are not assuming anything about the patient's personal life. It is just another indicated test
   d) HLA-B27 antibody test
      1) Recurrent non-granulomatous iritis with episodes of complete resolution in an otherwise healthy eye, and hyperacute iritis, are likely to be caused by HLA-B27
      2) A positive result explains the uveitis and changes your management by warning you to treat vigorously, taper slowly and expect recurrences
      3) It also indicates an inherited, non-specific predisposition to
         a) Uveitis
         b) Ankylosing spondylitis (lower back stiffness)
         c) Arthritis and juvenile rheumatoid arthritis
         d) Inflammatory bowel and Crohn's disease
         e) Psoriatic arthritis, psoriasis
         f) Other collagen vascular disorders
   e) Angiotensin converting enzyme (ACE): indicates pulmonary sarcoid only. Sarcoid is the leading cause of granulomatous iritis, especially in blacks and females
   f) Serum lysozyme: indicates non-pulmonary sarcoid. Localized inflammatory nodules can be found anywhere, including the uvea and conjunctiva; especially associated with granulomatous iritis, blacks, and females
   g) Antinuclear antibody (ANA): an autoimmune collagen vascular screen
      1) A positive result in a child probably indicates juvenile rheumatoid arthritis
      2) In an adult it probably indicates systemic lupus erythematosus
   h) Chest x-ray: to R/O pulmonary tuberculosis (TB) and sarcoid (ask about a persistent cough)
      1) Pulmonary TB lesions are necessary to cause uveitis

2) Pulmonary sarcoid lesions are not necessary to cause uveitis
3) Purified protein derivative (PPD) with anergy panel will test positive if there has ever been TB exposure, but if there are no lung lesions, it is not the cause of the uveitis
4) TB usually causes granulomatous KPs, but it may be difficult to determine

7) Expand the laboratory search based on uveitis questionnaire (see end of chapter) and exam findings
    a) Rheumatoid factor: rheumatoid arthritis is usually diagnosed long before it causes iritis. Order if
        1) Bad arthritis
        2) Scleritis
        3) Peripheral corneal thinning diseases. Also order anti-neutrophil cytoplasmic antibody (ANCA) test
    b) Conjunctival biopsy of nodules in recurrent granulomatous iritis: the only way to prove purely ocular sarcoid. Recommended for all granulomatous iritis, especially in blacks and females. Must be done before any systemic steroid use
    c) HLA-B5, another rare marker for a predisposition to iritis
    d) Behcet's skin puncture test: R/O Behcet's disease if Japanese or Mediterranean descent, hypopyon, retinal vasculitis, or bilateral with a history of mouth and urogenital sores. Get retina and internal medicine consults for this
    e) Crohn's or inflammatory bowel disease — recurrent diarrhea: no easy lab test, 10 – 20% have + HLA-B27, refer to family medical doctor or GI specialist for GI workup to R/O inflammatory bowel or Crohn's disease. You can manage the iritis conventionally
    f) Lyme titer and erythrocyte sedimentation rate (sed rate) and enzyme linked immuno absorbent assay (ELISA): if a history of a tick bite, fever, or rashes. Also order if pars planitis is present
    g) MRI of brain and orbits with thin sections through orbits to R/O demyelination from multiple sclerosis (MS): consider in females with paresthesia and a Hx of retrobulbar neuritis
    h) Juvenile rheumatoid arthritis: ANA and HLA-B8
    i) Reiter's syndrome: mostly a clinical diagnosis by an internist. Urethritis and uveitis followed by arthritis. May feature elevated HLA-B27 and various infectious diseases
    j) Tubulointerstitial nephritis and uveitis syndrome (TINU): an autoimmune disease causing kidney disease and usually bilateral, non-granulomatous anterior uveitis. The uveitis responds well to steroid therapy, though it may be recurrent or chronic. Order blood urea nitrogen (BUN), serum creatinine levels, sed rate, and urinalysis. Manage with a nephrologist

8) Iritis/uveitis syndromes that you should refer to a uveitis or retina specialist and the tests they may order

    a) Retinal vasculitis with oral or genital ulcers: HLA-B5, HLA-B57, HLA-B27 to R/O Behcet's (retina consult)

    b) Chorio-retinitis (if active, get a STAT retina consult): anti-toxoplasma, IgG, IgM to R/O toxo or histoplasmosis

    c) Retinal vasculitis and subacute sinus problems: ANCA test, chest x-ray, sinus CT, R/O Wegener's granulomatosis (retina consult)

    d) Choroiditis, exudative retinal detachment, tinnitus: fluorescein angiogram (FANG), audio testing, lumbar puncture, MRI, to R/O Harada's disease

    e) Vitritis in elderly female: vitreous biopsy to R/O lymphoma or infection

    f) Multifocal choroiditis of posterior pole in middle age males: HLA-A29 to R/O birdshot choroiditis

9) All of these tests are interpreted for you. The report will show the normal range and indicate your results. Abnormal results will be flagged

10) If history and exam results do not help focus your lab search, and the case meets criteria for further investigation, order a "shotgun panel"

UVEITIS QUESTIONNAIRE

Used with permission of F. Mitchel Opremcak, MD, The Ohio State University, Department of Ophthalmology

Family History

These questions refer to your grandparents, parents, aunts, uncles, brothers, sisters, children or grandchildren.

Has anyone in your **family** ever had

Tuberculosis	yes no
Syphilis	yes no
Arthritis or rheumatism	yes no
Diabetes	yes no
Allergies	yes no
Gout	yes no

Has anyone in your family had medical problems of the

Eyes	yes no
Skin	yes no
Kidneys	yes no
Lungs	yes no
Intestines	yes no
Brain	yes no

Social History

Have you lived out of the U.S.A.? Where?	yes no
Have you lived in other states? Where?	yes no
Is your job harmful to your eyes? How?	yes no
Have you ever owned a puppy?	yes no
Have you ever owned a cat?	yes no
Have you ever eaten raw meat or hamburger?	yes no
Do you drink untreated stream, well or lake water?	yes no
Have you ever been exposed to sick animals?	yes no
Do you smoke cigarettes?	yes no
Have you ever used IV drugs?	yes no
Have you ever had bisexual or homosexual relationships?	yes no
Have you ever taken birth control pills?	yes no

Personal Medical History

Have **you** ever had the following diseases?

Anemia	yes no
Cancer	yes no
Diabetes	yes no
Hepatitis	yes no
High BP	yes no
Pleurisy	yes no
Pneumonia	yes no
Ulcers	yes no
Herpes	yes no
Chicken pox	yes no
Shingles or Zoster	yes no
German measles or Rubella	yes no
Mumps	yes no
Chlamydia or Trachoma	yes no
Syphilis	yes no
Gonorrhea	yes no
Tuberculosis (TB)	yes no
Leprosy	yes no
Leptospirosis	yes no
Histoplasmosis	yes no
Candida or Moniliasis fungal infection	yes no
Coccidiomycosis	yes no
Sporotrichosis	yes no
Cryptococcal infection	yes no
Toxoplasmosis	yes no
Amoeba infection	yes no
Giardiasis	yes no
Toxocariasis	yes no
Cysticercosis	yes no
Trichinosis	yes no
Whipple's disease	yes no
Hay fever	yes no
Allergies	yes no
Pemphigoid	yes no
Vasculitis	yes no
Rheumatoid arthritis	yes no
Arthritis	yes no
Lupus or systemic lupus erythematosus	yes no
Scleroderma	yes no
Reiter's syndrome	yes no
Colitis	yes no
Psoriasis	yes no
Behcet's disease	yes no
Temporal arteritis	yes no
Erythema nodosa	yes no
Multiple sclerosis	yes no

Sarcoid   yes no

Have you ever had any of the following symptoms?

General Health

Chills   yes no
Fevers (persistent or recurrent)   yes no
Night sweats   yes no
Fatigue or tire easily   yes no
Poor appetite   yes no
Recent weight loss   yes no
Do you consider yourself to be sick?   yes no

Head

Frequent or severe headaches   yes no
Frequent or severe dizziness   yes no
Fainting   yes no
Numbness or tingling in your body   yes no
Paralysis in parts of your body   yes no
Seizures or convulsions   yes no

Nose and Throat

Sores in your nose or mouth   yes no
Severe or recurrent nosebleeds   yes no
Frequent sneezing   yes no
Sinus problems   yes no
Persistent hoarseness   yes no
Tooth or gum infections   yes no
Sore throat   yes no
Dry mouth   yes no

Skin

Rashes   yes no
Skin sores   yes no
Sunburn easily (photosensitivity)   yes no
White patches of skin or hair   yes no
Tick or insect bites   yes no
Painfully cold fingers   yes no
Severe itching   yes no

Respiratory

Severe or frequent colds   yes no
Constant coughing   yes no
Coughing up blood   yes no

Pneumonia   yes no
Recent flu or viral infection   yes no
Wheezing   yes no

Blood

Frequent or easy bruising   yes no
Frequent or easy bleeding   yes no
Shortness of breath   yes no
Blood transfusion   yes no

Gastrointestinal

Diarrhea   yes no
Bloody stools   yes no
Severe heartburn or ulcers   yes no
Jaundice or yellow skin   yes no

Bones and Joints

Stiff joints   yes no
Painful joints   yes no
Swollen joints   yes no
Red and hot joints   yes no
Stiff lower back   yes no
Back pain while sleeping   yes no
Neuralgia   yes no
Muscle aches   yes no

Genitourinary

Kidney problems   yes no
Bladder problems   yes no
Blood in your urine   yes no
Urinary discharge   yes no
Genital sores or ulcers   yes no
Prostate problems   yes no
Testicular pain   yes no
Are you pregnant or plan to be?   yes no

What is your present weight? ___________
What is your present height? ___________

____
Signature   Date

Notes

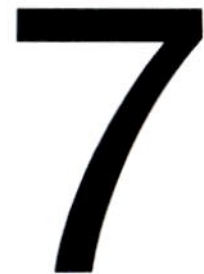

ACUTE ANGLE CLOSURE GLAUCOMA

A) Subjective
1) Pain, redness
2) Blur, halos, nausea, vomiting may not be present with lower pressures

B) Objective
1) Acutely elevated IOP
2) Epithelial microcystic edema if very high acute IOP increase
3) Fixed, mid-dilated pupil
4) Closed angle via Van Herrick
5) Cupping is not diagnostic. Pallor is usually present
6) Do gonioscopy; glycerin will clear the cornea if necessary. Use anesthetic first
7) Other findings depend on etiology (*e.g.*, hyperopia, trauma, intumescent cataract, aniridia, neovascularization of the iris, etc.)

C) Assessment
1) Acute high IOP can exist with an open angle
2) Look for inflammation, pigment, or heme in the AC
3) R/O iris neovascularization and peripheral anterior synechiae

D) Plan
1) Pilocarpine 2%: may not be effective until the IOP is <50. It will pull the iris out of the angle allowing drainage. Use pilocarpine with caution in aphakes or pseudophakes
2) Compress while doing gonioscopy with a 4-mirror gonio lens. Try to push the iris back to open the angle. Push/release in 30 sec cycles until the angle stays open or the IOP is down
3) Instill all available glaucoma drops (beta blocker if no contraindication, Azopt or Trusopt, prostaglandin) and Pred Forte multiple times
4) Isosorbide: if unable to open the angle with 4-mirror gonio pressure, the patient is in good cardiovascular health, no nausea, and topical treatment is not working, administer 1.5 grams per kilogram of 45% isosorbide over ice
5) Pounds - 10% ÷ 2 = kilograms

6) Confirm the angle is open and maintain the patient on pilocarpine qid until a peripheral iridectomy is done
7) Treat any other underlying problem

Notes

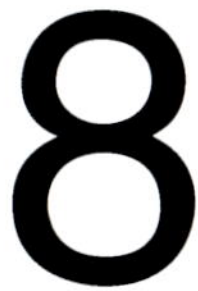

GLAUCOMA — LONG TERM MANAGEMENT

A) Subjective: usually no subjective signs or symptoms

B) Objective
1) Age: treat younger patients more aggressively (lower target pressure). They will probably gradually lose some field regardless
   a) 0.1% incidence in Australians 40 – 45 yrs old
   b) 10% incidence in Australians >80 yrs old
2) Race: treat black patients more aggressively. They are 4x more likely to develop glaucoma than whites and are more likely to progress
3) Medical history
   a) Encourage compliance in treating cardiovascular diseases such as diabetes, hypertension, high cholesterol, heart disease, etc.
   b) Systemic beta blockers will cause 2 – 4 mmHg IOP lowering and may make topical beta blockers ineffective. The IOP can go up if a systemic beta blocker is discontinued
   c) History of significant blood loss (bleeding ulcer or major surgery) can account for optic nerve damage. Treat as possible low tension glaucoma (LTG), and monitor nerve and fields for progression to determine goal IOP
   d) History of migraine is a risk factor for LTG
4) Family history
   a) How many family members have glaucoma? Maternal Hx is worse. A 10% risk of primary open angle glaucoma (POAG) if close relatives have it (4x – 8x increased risk)
   b) At what age did they develop glaucoma?
   c) Did they have LTG? Indicates increased risk
5) IOP
   a) Find out pretreatment IOPs
   b) Start a glaucoma flow sheet listing dates, IOPs, CDs, meds used
   c) Set initial target IOPs; some rules of thumb
      1) LTG with pretreatment IOP in mid teens: goal 8 – 12
      2) Advanced POAG field loss and <0.1 rim or notched out, goal: low teens (10 – 13)

       3) Moderately advanced POAG field loss and at least a 0.1 rim through 360°, goal <15
       4) Common early POAG, goal = 18
       5) Ocular hypertension or POAG with pretreatment IOP 28 or higher, goal = 21
   d) In one major study of primary open angle glaucoma, no patients with stable IOP ≤ 14 mmHg progressed. 4% of those with IOPs ≤ 17 had progression
   e) Update and lower target IOPs by at least 2 – 3 mm if
       1) Increasing CDs according to stereo photos or careful disk drawings
       2) Confirmed field progression (repeat)
   f) Do serial tonometry to get a reliable baseline: a variable high IOP is more damaging than a stable high IOP
       1) Initially if LTG
       2) Initially if variable IOP Hx
       3) If you later question the accuracy of the glaucoma diagnosis, or the efficacy of medications, stop drops for 2 weeks and do serial IOP
       4) If fields or nerves progressively deteriorate despite meeting target IOP, do serial tonometry while on medications
       5) Take the first IOP by 8:00 a.m. if possible, then every 1 – 2 hrs until the end of the day. To bill serial tonometry you need 5 readings.
   g) Get accurate, reproducible applanation readings. No other method is acceptable for treating glaucoma
       1) Align tonometer axis with corneal toricity if it is highly toric
       2) Ask the patient to breathe normally and relax
       3) Measure right eye (OD), left eye (OS), OD; if OD readings are consistent, stop; if subsequent readings are lower, keep repeating measurements until consistent
       4) A 10% or 2 mm error is possible with a single reading. Repeat until consistent, then allow 1 – 2 mm variance from goal IOP
       5) Most error factors artificially elevate readings. Your lowest reading is usually the accurate one
       6) Corneal thinning such as caused by excimer laser refractive surgery lowers applanation readings by approximately 3 mmHG
       7) Goldmann tonometer calibrated for a 520 micron cornea. Pachymetry is very helpful here
          a) For each 20 microns >520, reduce your reading by 1 mmHg for true IOP
          b) For each 20 microns <520, increase your reading by 1 mmHg for true IOP
6) Gonioscopy
   a) Do initially as part of a glaucoma workup and yearly thereafter

    b) Be sure the angle is not occluded or occludable. Record the most posterior structure seen without depressing the cornea

    c) A Posner lens is less likely to cause striae in the cornea while viewing than a Zeiss lens. A Goldmann lens should give the truest view of the angle but takes longer

    d) Only the posterior half of the trabecular meshwork drains aqueous

    e) Record the amount of pigment in the meshwork

    f) Heavy pigment with a concave iris may be a clue to pigment dispersion caused by a reverse pupil block. This may be treated with a peripheral iridectomy if <age 40

    g) Look for pigment clumping, inflammatory debris and exfoliative debris in inferior angle

    h) Look carefully for rubeosis if there is a history of diabetes or vein occlusion

    i) Look for angle recession if a history of ocular trauma

    j) Repeat yearly; initially open angles can close over time and cause combined mechanism glaucoma

    k) Do after applanation; it only takes a minute with a Zeiss or Posner (the cornea is already anesthetized)

7) Monitor optic nerves carefully

    a) Recommend 90 D or 78 D fundus lens

    b) Contact lens or gonio lens view is also excellent

    c) Direct and binocular indirect ophthalmoscope (BIO) view is not acceptable to treat glaucoma

    d) Do not use Superfield or 60 D unless you are aware when you lose binocularity. These lenses need a large dilation to get binocularity, often impossible in elderly. When viewing binocularily they give an enhanced view of depth and contour

    e) Catching nerve head changes is most important in ocular hypertension and early glaucoma when the nerve is relatively healthy and there is not enough damage to cause a visual field defect for your perimeter to track

    f) Stereo photos highly recommended

        1) Nidek stereo photos are best, standardized, enhanced stereopsis

        2) 35 mm stereo slides or digital photos also good; need a stereo viewer

        3) Non-myd and Polaroid cameras do not have enough resolution

        4) Repeat photos when the disk changes

        5) Progression of peripapillary atrophy indicates glaucoma progression

    g) Disk drawings are necessary, especially if you have no camera

        1) Recommend a 10x10 grid circle, stamp or preprinted

        2) Record horizontal and vertical CD on all routine exams

        3) If CD >0.7, look at the rim, not the cup

       4) Memorize the rim thickness at the actual 12:00, 3:00, 6:00, and 9:00. Then mark your grid at those locations. Sketch the cup margin, note pallor and slope. Draw contour. Do not be fooled by color change. Use stereopsis to see the edge; search the rim methodically

       5) ISNT rule: in a healthy optic nerve the inferior rim is usually thickest, followed by the superior, nasal, and the temporal rim is the thinnest

       6) Consider a direct ophthalmoscopy view at each IOP check to catch disk hemorrhages. Assuming no other causes such as diabetes or vein occlusion, hemorrhages may indicate progression of the glaucoma. Lower the IOP if feasible; watch for a future notch and field loss here

  h) Nerve fiber layer analysis

       1) Use a direct ophthalmoscope with a red free filter

       2) Look for a darker, slit shape defect in the shiny superior and inferior NFL reflection or a relative difference in appearance between superior and inferior NFL

       3) Very difficult, clear media are necessary

       4) Get an automated nerve fiber layer analysis done if in doubt and you need the information to make the diagnosis

  i) Computerized nerve head and nerve fiber layer analysis: in early questionable glaucoma, access to an automated nerve fiber layer analyzer can be valuable. Once the field loss is established, careful visual fields are the most accurate way to follow progression. In advanced age or senility, yearly nerve fiber analysis may have to take the place of yearly fields

  j) Estimate nerve size: a 0.7 cup in a small nerve is more significant than a 0.7 cup in a large nerve. This information is very helpful in borderline cases

       1) Direct ophthalmoscopy

          a) Shine spot on the nerve head with a dilated pupil

          b) Record nerve size as normal or as a percentage of normal size

          c) Sizes usually range from 80% – 130% of normal size

       2) Indirect ophthalmoscopy

          a) Use a 66 D superfield lens

          b) Adjust the width of your beam to match the width of the nerve head

          c) Read the scale for the beam width on the slit lamp

          d) 1 mm = 1000 microns (very small)
             1.5 mm = 1500 microns (normal)
             2.0 mm = 2000 microns (very large)

       3) Very useful in making the initial diagnosis in borderline cases

  k) Peripapillary atrophy is a minor risk factor, but progression of atrophy may be a sign of glaucoma progression

8) Automated visual fields

a) FDT or Matrix: frequency doubling technology by Humphrey-Zeiss
   1) An effective, rapid visual field screener
   2) Not a substitute for traditional automated fields when diagnosing or following glaucoma
   3) Can miss small scotomas
b) Humphrey-Zeiss (see Chapter 9)
   1) Fovea thresholds are important for long term care
   2) Overview and statistical analysis are best for long term care
   3) Humphrey is the dominant field analyzer
   4) It is not important that all medical doctors use Humphrey. It may be important to use what your glaucoma tertiary care doctor uses so you can directly compare fields
   5) Humphrey Field Analyzer II (HFA II) is worth upgrading to if you need a new machine because of new features
      a) Swedish interactive thresholding algorithm (SITA Standard): the new standard of care
         1) ½ the time of a full threshold
         2) Defects show as less deep
         3) Probably represents visual function better than a full threshold because of less fatigue
      b) SITA Fast
         1) Takes about as long as a screening field, but it gives some threshold information for the elderly or inattentive
         2) It is not acceptable to use for routine glaucoma care
      c) Short wavelength automated perimetry (SWAP) (blue-yellow) perimetry can detect field loss earlier, but
         1) A very difficult test for patients to take. Use only on experienced alert patients with clear media
         2) Ignore mild defects because of false positives. A cluster of 4 points at P<5% or 3 points at P<1% yield sensitivity of 95% and specificity of 75%
         3) Repeat the test to increase confidence
   6) If you have a series of fields on a patient and you are worried about possible deterioration, repeat the same strategy for an apples to apples comparison. If you are confident the patient is stable, you can perform a SITA Standard for a new baseline, but expect the defects to be less deep. Humphrey claims the SITA result is actually a more accurate representation of the visual field
   7) Recommendations
      a) 24-2 SITA Standard with fovea threshold: use on new glaucoma patients if time is a concern, 7 min
      b) 30-2 SITA Standard with fovea: use for suspected central nervous system disorders. Best for glaucoma in case the scotoma goes to the edge of a 24-2 field and other conditions, 9 min

      c) 24-2 SITA Fast without fovea threshold: no fluctuation data and less reliability. Use only when the patient is unable to do a longer test, 4 min

      d) Choose a size V stimulus in advanced glaucoma when the field is mostly blacked out

      e) Choose a central 10° field when that is all that is left or if there is paracentral loss so you can more closely track changes

      f) Monitor fovea threshold, Snellen acuity, and count finger vision depending on the severity of the loss. Glaucoma does affect central vision eventually

      g) Ask the patient how his/her vision is doing. Patients can tell when they are progressing in late stage disease

   8) Write up instructions for dilation, lenses, strategy, etc. for staff

   9) Do visual field (VF) interpretation, assessment, plan. Write interpretation in the chart. Describe the field loss and whether it is stable or progressing. Bill evaluations and management (E&M) if you do examine the patient (see Appendix — Medical Coding), and VF

C) Assessment

   1) Review the total picture once a yr or whenever you suspect progression

      a) Pretreatment IOP, treatment IOP, and current IOP

      b) Pretreatment nerve appearance, progression, current nerve appearance

      c) Pretreatment visual fields, progression, and latest field

      d) Is the angle closing and causing combined mechanism glaucoma?

      e) Has the patient's general health changed substantially?

      f) Review drop instillation

      g) Review compliance

      h) Review side effects

   2) What is the patient's life expectancy versus the rate of vision loss? We all lose some function naturally as we age (0.1 decibel (db) of mean deviation per yr)

   3) Consider the benefit of very aggressive therapy versus the cost in time, money and quality of life for the patient. Take into consideration the patient's life expectancy

   4) When treating with multiple medications, consider stopping one or more of them to see if they are still effective

   5) Always ask about side effects from the medications

   6) Always set a new target IOP when you do a DFE or at least once a yr

   7) You need to consider that there is a high risk of progression of vision loss with treated POAG over long periods of time

      a) After 20 yrs of treatment, a 27% probability of legal blindness in one eye and a 9% probability of blindness in both eyes

      b) Twice as many cases of blindness are due to visual field criteria as are due to central acuity loss. Patients are not functionally impaired by peripheral loss as much as by central loss
8) Risk analysis by Graham
    a) Ocular hypertension risk analysis by Graham
      1) Risk factors are thin corneas, large CD, IOP, age
      2) Non-treated, 9.5% progress
      3) Treated, 4.4% progress
    b) LTG
      1) Risk factors are female sex, migraine Hx, disk hemorrhages
      2) Non-treated, 60% progress
      3) Treated, 20% progress
    c) Early glaucoma
      1) Risk factors are exfoliation, IOP, VF loss, age, disk hemorrhages
      2) Non-treated, 62% progress
      3) Treated, 45% progress
    d) Advanced glaucoma
      1) Risk factors are IOP, age, IOP fluctuation
      2) Non-treated, no data
      3) Treated, 30% progress

D) Plan

1) POAG medications: we do not "treat glaucoma," we treat a risk factor: pressures
    a) First line medications: prostaglandins
      1) Xalatan 0.005% (Lumigan 0.03%, Travatan 0.004%), Travatan Z 0.004% (no BAK preservative)
        a) Qhs dosing helps compliance
        b) Very effective, 25% – 30% IOP drop in patients for whom the drug is effective
        c) These drugs are best at flattening the diurnal curve
        d) Travatan: more effective in blacks
        e) Warn about possible iris changes, especially in a hazel iris
        f) Rare thickening and pigmentation of lashes
        g) Iritis and CME also possible, but usually with preexisting risk factors such as pseudophakia, aphakia, a compromised retina, history of iritis, or recent eye surgery
        h) May take >1 month to reach full effectiveness
        i) Theoretically not additive with Pilo, but actually works sometimes
        j) Due to uveo-scleral outflow mechanism of action, lower pressures are possible when treating LTG

    2) Beta blockers have a longer track record, but must be used with caution in patients with heart or lung problems. Expect about a 25% IOP drop. Most require bid dosing
        a) Cardioselective, less IOP drop but better nerve micro circulation in LTG
            1) Betoptic S 0.25% (shake) preferred
        b) Once a day dosing; use in the a.m. is more effective
            1) Timoptic XE 0.25% and 0.5%
            2) Betagan 0.25% and 0.5%
        c) Neuroprotective? Less nocturnal systemic hypotension and less decrease in "good" HDL
            1) Ocupress 1.0%
            2) Betoptic S 0.25%
        d) The rest: (Who will give you samples?)
            1) Timoptic 0.25% and 0.5%
            2) OptiPranolol 0.3%
            3) Generics
            4) Put p.m. dose in at supper time so hypotensive side effects can be noticed
  b) Second line drugs
    1) Trusopt 2%, Azopt
        a) Topical versions of carbonic anhydrase inhibitors work about as well, without the side effects
        b) Approximately 16 – 20% IOP drop
        c) Bid gives as much effect as the recommended tid unless a dark iris color
        d) Azopt should sting less, less expensive
    2) Alphagan P 0.15%
        a) A less toxic and less allergenic form of Iopidine
        b) Bid as effective as tid
        c) Approximately a 20% IOP drop expected
        d) May be neuroprotective
        e) Do not use <age 2 or in pregnant mothers. Alphagan crosses the blood-brain barrier easily in kids and can cause death
    3) Cosopt bid: combination of 0.5% Timoptic and Trusopt 2%, very useful and potent. Could also combine with Alphagan if needed for neuroprotective effect
    4) Combigan: combination of Alphagan 0.2% and timolol 0.5%, bid dosing
    5) Xalcom: combination of 0.005% Xalatan and timolol 0.5% maleate. Once per day dosing, time so peak effect of timolol covers the diurnal peak. Available soon
    6) Extravan: combination of travoprost 0.004% and timolol 0.5%. Available soon
  c) Third line drugs
    1) Pilocarpine drops 1% – 4%
        a) A last medical resort, but they are very effective and the symptoms are usually well tolerated in the elderly

        b) Warn about miosis, brow ache, retinal detachment Sx
        c) Tid dosing with punctal occlusion works as well as qid
        d) Have the patient discontinue 2 days before a yearly
           dilated fundus exam
        e) Inexpensive
      2) Pilopine HS gel or Ocusert
        a) Hs dosing is a more practical alternative for many
    d) Limited value drugs
      1) Epinephrine
      2) Propine
      3) Carbachol
      4) Iopidine
      5) Echothiophate Iodide
      6) Diamox and Neptazane (except for angle closure)

2) Strategy
    a) All glaucoma meds will fail in about 15% of patients due to
      ineffectiveness or allergy
    b) Unless IOPs are very stable and reliable, start all new
      medications with a uniocular trial
    c) Expect a 2 mm crossover effect with beta blockers
    d) Give a sample to establish the efficacy of the drug before
      asking the patient to pay $20 – $80 for a bottle that may not
      work. RTC in 3 weeks before the sample runs out
    e) If 1 drop only gives a minimal effect, stop it before trying
      another
    f) Consider Timoptic XE or Betagan qam and Xalatan qhs for
      combination convenience
    g) Cosopt or Combigan with a prostaglandin analog gives 3
      powerful medications in 2 drops

3) LTG: special considerations
    a) Prostaglandin analogs: will give the lowest pressure with no
      BP effect
    b) Alphagan: possible neuroprotective effect and no lipid effect
    c) Ocupress and Betoptic S: possible neuroprotective effect
    d) Consider asking family medical doctor to Rx an oral calcium
      channel blocker to help nerve head perfusion
    e) Exercise may be helpful to reduce IOP as well as being good
      for circulation
    f) Ginkgo biloba may increase perfusion of nerve head

4) Argon laser trabeculoplasty (ALT) or selective laser
  trabeculoplasty (SLT)
    a) SLT is newer and has the advantage of being repeatable and
      less damaging to the meshwork
    b) Consider whenever compliance is a problem or the patient
      needs 3 or more drops to achieve target IOP
    c) Less effective in angle recession
    d) The biggest risk is a post-op IOP spike that Iopidine usually
      controls well

   e) All current glaucoma meds are continued for 1 month, then try
      tapering back medications
   f) ALT is equal in effect to about 1 topical medication
   g) Steroid qid is typically prescribed
   h) Taper the steroid after 3 – 4 days
5) Trabeculectomy with mitomycin C: hands-on experience with the
   surgeon is recommended before doing immediate post-op care
   a) 70 – 80% success rate
   b) All glaucoma meds should have been discontinued initially
      after surgery, though they may be added back later
   c) Goals of 8 – 12 mmHg are usually possible
   d) Careful post-op follow up necessary to ensure good bleb
      formation and filtration
      1) R/O Seidel's sign
      2) Bleb should be medium or large size
      3) Bleb should be avascular or mildly vascular
      4) Bleb should have elevation or a bubble formation
      5) Microcysts should be visible on about 50% of the surface
         of the bleb
   e) If the IOP rises and the above 5 factors are not present, action
      is needed to save the bleb
      1) If a releasable suture was placed, remove it and see if the
         IOP decreases
      2) Apply digital pressure in 10 sec increments to reduce the
         IOP to about 10
         a) Have the patient look up
         b) Push against the lower lid with your finger to raise the
            IOP to an estimated 40 – 50 mmHg for 2 sec
         c) Remeasure the IOP
         d) The bleb should be fuller looking and increase in size
         e) Repeat as necessary to lower the IOP to the low teens
      3) Increase topical steroids
      4) When the bleb is functioning properly, more of the above 5
         factors will be present and the IOP will be lower
      5) Some patients need to do home digital pressure
      6) Blebitis can rapidly lead to endophthalmitis. If blebitis is
         suspected, call the surgeon, culture, and start on 4th
         generation fluoroquinolone drops. Watch for these signs
         a) Vascular bleb
         b) Mild iritis
         c) Pus or WBC in the bleb
         d) Discomfort
      7) Always look for choroidal folds and worry about Seidel's
         sign and endophthalmitis. Continue topical antibiotics
         through the post-op period
      8) Once the patient and the bleb are stable, there is low risk
         in comanaging if you keep the above points in mind
      9) Trabeculectomy with mitomycin-C gives excellent long
         term reduction of IOP. Hypotony (IOP <6 mmHg) occurs in

approximately 40% of eyes within 2 yrs, however. The incidence of hypotony maculopathy is about 9%. Younger whites are at greater risk for hypotony

10) Trabeculectomy accelerates cataract development

Notes____

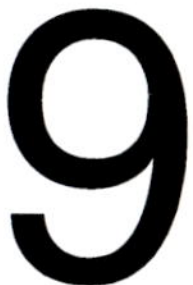

ADVANCED INTERPRETATION OF
HUMPHREY VISUAL FIELDS IN GLAUCOMA

A) Choose the size of field
1) 24-2 is about 2 min faster than 30-2
2) 30-2 recommended for glaucoma, neurologic, optic nerve problems. The extra peripheral points may help distinguish an arcuate scotoma from a lid artifact if there is a normal point peripheral to the scotoma
3) 10-2 use for end stage glaucoma when all other periphery is lost or for low tension glaucoma (LTG) with paracentral loss. Also use if plotting macular disease

B) Choose a strategy
1) Full "4-2" threshold dims target in increments of 4 db until no longer seen, then brightens in 2 db increments. Was the gold standard, but is brutal on patients, especially if doing 30-2. It is actually less accurate for many patients due to fatigue
2) FastPac uses 3 db steps to cross the threshold once. Faster but less precise
3) Swedish interactive thresholding algorithm (SITA) Standard: artificial intelligence that reprocesses "4-2" staircase strategies. Available on the Humphrey Field Analyzer II (HFA II) only
    a) Speed of presentation changes according to reaction time
    b) Makes assumptions about a point based on age-normal
    c) Once 1 point is tested, it can make assumptions about the starting brightness to test adjacent points
    d) Test questions are modified according to frequency of seeing responses and false responses
    e) Quits testing a point when statistically satisfied that it has an accurate result. May retest later if an adjacent point result changes its confidence about the earlier point
    f) Uses all information from all points, not just the last stimulus to cross the threshold
    g) Does not retest points to get reliability; it calculates mathematically
    h) Does not measure short term fluctuation; not worth the time

i) Reduces 24-2 and 30-2 test time by 50% from full threshold times

j) Depths of defects will be less than on full threshold; Humphrey claims it is actually more accurate due to less fatigue

k) Early defects found with full threshold may not appear with SITA; they are artifacts due to fatigue

l) Used by glaucoma specialists. Use it for all new fields and stable old fields when a strict comparison is not necessary

4) SITA Fast is very fast, about 4 min. Use as a screening field and on very inattentive patients. It gives some threshold information but is not acceptable for routine glaucoma diagnosis or treatment because it misses many scotomas. On HFA II only

5) If detection of change is critical, use the same strategy as used before!

6) SITA and SITA Fast can be used with a 10-2 and blue-yellow field, but not with a size 5

C) Choose a target

1) The default is size 3 white on white for statistical comparisons

2) Use size 5 when size 3 fields are going black, but no statistical references are given

3) Short wavelength automated perimetry (SWAP) (blue-yellow)

    a) Gives false positive clutter and is very difficult for patient

    b) Turn off short term fluctuation

    c) Claimed 2 – 5 yrs sooner detection of glaucoma field loss because it isolates a pathway that has less redundancy and damage is easier to detect

    d) Use only on good, experienced field takers with clear media. Warn patients about strange effects. The target may be seen as an achromatic or violet colored sensation

    e) Use on patients when you really want to treat but you need one more justification. Do not run on all 0.6 CD's who pass a white/white field

D) Set up test

1) Dilate if <3 mm pupil or cataracts are present

2) Use full diameter style trial lenses

3) Dim the room while setting up the machine to allow the first eye to dark adapt

4) Use the fovea threshold on almost all patients; it is handy information to have and to track long term

5) Turn on the reliability test function

6) Use a white eye patch to preserve sensitivity in the second eye

7) HFA II allows customized buttons to set up your favorite test variables for convenience

8) Consider turning off gaze tracker if a technician monitors; will save time and trouble

E) Run test
1) Have a good technician in room explaining, giving encouragement and feedback
2) Remember to tell the patient to pause the test by holding the clicker down, if needed
3) Test a severely damaged eye last
4) Turn the nose out of the way
5) Place the lens close
6) Tape the lid if necessary
7) Recognize fixation and reliability problems as they occur and correct them then
8) The technician needs to write an impression of fixation, reliability and any unusual problems on the printout

F) Print test
1) If non-standard parameters (size 5, central 10-2, or blue-yellow) are used, the only option is the 3-in-1 (grey scale, depth of defect, and actual threshold in db). No statistical analysis is available
2) If 30-2 and 24-2 size with any threshold strategy print the Single Field Analysis for statistical analysis
3) If this is the second or greater set of fields for this patient also select Overview and Change Analysis. You can now weed out all old field copies from the record

G) Interpret single field analysis: "How are the fields today?"
1) Glance at the grey scale first. Admit it, we all do!
   a) Greyness is smoothed or interpolated between points
   b) Darker grey is not necessarily abnormal
2) Check reliability factors
   a) Read technician's impression of fixation and reliability
   b) Fixation losses (from checking blind spot) should be less than 20% or HFA will flag with xx and print "low patient reliability"
   c) False positives (makes a noise and pauses to catch happy clickers) should be less than 15% or HFA flags with xx
   d) False negatives (shows a light 9 db brighter than threshold at a previously tested point) are flagged with xx if calculated to be abnormal. These values rise in advanced glaucoma
   e) If the patient has reduced reliability, but the probability plots show a normal field, statistically the field is probably normal. But if the probability plots show a defect, you must repeat the test
3) Decibel plot (the actual result for each tested point). With a full threshold you can look at tested and retested points (in parentheses) and compare for reliability
4) Total deviation measures defects in patient's hill of vision compared to an age-matched normal hill of vision. Compensates for loss of sensitivity toward periphery
   a) A general reduction in vision such as caused by a cataract will give a lot of false positive results

   b) If a patient has better than average overall sensitivity (such as a pseudophake whose age-matched peer group all had lens opacities) this will pick up an earlier relative defect
   c) Plots show a <5%, <2%, <1%, or <½% chance that a normal age-matched person would have that threshold result at that point
 5) Pattern deviation starts with total deviation and adjusts for overall loss of sensitivity such as cataract or refractive error
   a) Glaucoma visual field analysis is usually pattern recognition
   b) This is usually most valuable plot because it allows the pattern to show through
   c) Watch for any defect that respects the midline. This indicates a likely neurologic problem that should be investigated with MRI
 6) Glaucoma hemifield test (GHT)
   a) Compares 5 clusters of points above vs. below the midline
   b) The computer judges the field as Normal, Outside Normal Limits, Borderline, General Reduction of Sensitivity, or Abnormally High Sensitivity (happy clickers)
   c) Very useful, but not as sensitive as an experienced practitioner with good pattern recognition skills who knows what the nerve looks like
   d) Not available with FastPac
 7) Mean deviation (MD)
   a) Shows in db the overall sensitivity (height of hill of vision) compared to age-matched normal
   b) A positive number means better than normal sensitivity
   c) A negative number means worse than average
   d) If no probability given, then in a normal range
   e) The probability that a healthy age-matched patient would have this result is listed if significant
   f) More useful in advanced glaucoma
 8) Pattern standard deviation (PSD)
   a) A normal hill of vision has smooth slopes. This would give a lower number result
   b) A rough hill of vision is more likely to be pathologic and will be flagged with a P value
   c) Not very useful on a single analysis
   d) Gets worse in early glaucoma then improves in late glaucoma. The hill gets smoother as it flat-lines! Also occurs in CPSD (see below)
   e) Very useful when used as comparison
 9) Short term fluctuation (SF): not in SITA
   a) Calculated from the 10 double thresholded points if you turned on the short term fluctuation option. Not done with SITA
   b) If abnormal, flagged with a P value
   c) Important as a measure of reliability
   d) Fluctuation increases in moderately advanced glaucoma
 10) Corrected pattern standard deviation (CPSD): not in SITA

a) Same as PSD but corrected for age and short term fluctuation

H) Interpret overview: "Seeing the forest and not just trees." Using your pattern recognition, you can recognize stable or deteriorating fields without flipping through a thick chart
1) Look at grey scales in chronological order
    a) Even though grey scales can mislead when used as a one time analysis, it is valid to look for trends or change if the same strategy was used
    b) If 24-2 and 30-2 fields are mixed, don't be fooled by peripheral darkness on the 30-2 that is not presented on 24-2 fields
    c) Check pupil sizes to see if they were consistent and that proper corrective lenses were used
2) Threshold values in db
    a) Give exact numbers to compare defects over time
    b) Use to confirm suspicions raised by other analysis
        1) Media, pupils, attentiveness and your test strategy can change over time
        2) Usually too much variability in the test for reliable direct comparison of individual points
3) Total deviation — important
    a) Scan vertically in order to look for changes and trends in pattern
4) Pattern deviation — most important!
    a) Scan vertically
    b) Easy to see change when you have 10 or 15 fields to look at!
5) Fovea threshold
    a) Very nice to have, especially in patients with advanced disease
6) MD, PSD, SF, and CPSD
    a) All are available if you want to compare sequentially, but hard to spot trends here

I) Interpret change analysis: "The trend is your friend"
1) Box plots: an excellent tool for spotting trends in long term patients!
    a) Histograms summarize differences between your patient's results and age-matched normals
    b) "Normal patient" plotted to the left
    c) Dates are listed
    d) Look at the average field sensitivity: should stay about level
    e) Look at the slope of the upper end of the box (85th percentile)
    f) Look at the slope of the lower end of the box (15th percentile)
    g) Are the boxes getting more compact (learning curve)?
    h) Are the boxes getting taller (more pattern deviation or increasing depth of localized field loss)?
    i) Look at top and bottom tails (best and worst 15% of points in the fields). Less useful, they only show very localized defects
2) SF: not in SITA

a) Should initially improve with learning curve
b) Will worsen as glaucoma progresses; more variability
c) Note lines showing where 5% and 1% probability of normality are, but the trend is more important (also used on the remaining statistical analysis)
d) Note the explanation of symbols to left highlighting results with reduced reliability from FastPac

3) MD
a) Shows the trend of the overall sensitivity of vision
b) Shows overall failing vision in late disease, but not much help following early localized disease

4) PSD
a) Shows the trend in the irregularity of the hill of vision
b) Remember that in late glaucoma the CPSD improves because the hill of vision is less rough as it flat-lines!

5) CPSD: not in SITA
a) Pattern standard deviation corrected for short term fluctuation
b) On full threshold only

6) MD slope
a) Mean deviation slope calculated with linear regression analysis when you have >5 fields
b) Normals lose 0.1 db per yr or 1 db per decade
c) Significance calculated with P value

Notes ____

____

____

____

____

____

____

____

____

____

____

____

____

____

10

AGE RELATED MACULAR DEGENERATION

A) Subjective
1) Painless, monocular or binocular loss of vision
2) Usually gradual onset, though a sudden loss in one eye could indicate exudative age related macular degeneration (ARMD)
3) History of smoking, obesity, white race, or high UV exposure are risk factors

B) Objective
1) VA and pinhole or best corrected VA
2) Pupils: normal
3) Confrontation fields: normal
4) BP: cardiovascular problems can contribute to ARMD
5) Extraocular eye movements: normal
6) External and slit lamp: normal
7) Amsler grid testing: may be normal in early stages but abnormal in later stages
8) DFE with fundus lens or contact lens
   a) Drusen in the macular area: either hard yellow drusen or larger soft drusen
   b) Retinal pigment epithelium loss or clumping: from small drop-out lesions to large geographic areas
   c) Epiretinal membranes may be present
      1) Appear as a shiny, wrinkled "cellophane" membrane lying on the surface of the macula
      2) The membrane may cause traction and lead to visible wrinkles in the macula and macular holes or pseudoholes
   d) Choroidal neovascular membrane (CNVM) signs
      1) A dirty gray-green membrane under the retina
      2) Subretinal macular hemorrhage
      3) Subretinal macular exudates
      4) Subretinal pigment ring
      5) A disciform scar may be present in late disease
      6) In some cases there may be no visible sign and a FANG and/or an indocyanine green (ICG) test must be done if the symptoms are strong

C) Assessment
   1) Amsler grid distortions are more likely in exudative ARMD
   2) When in doubt, do a careful stereoscopic evaluation of the macula
      with a contact lens, looking for any sign of neovascular
      membranes, leakage, exudation or thickening
   3) Hard drusen are a risk factor for wet ARMD
   4) Soft drusen are a **high** risk factor for wet ARMD
   5) ARMD is a risk indicator for poorer survival in women (not men)

D) Plan
   1) If wet or exudative ARMD cannot be ruled out
      a) Order an urgent FANG and retina consult
      b) The retina specialist may also order an ICG if the CNVM is
         occult and cannot be localized with fluorescein angiography
      c) A neovascular net can progress from treatable to untreatable
         in days
      d) Photodynamic therapy and intra-ocular injectables allow
         sealing of leaking vessels that were previously untreatable
   2) Dry ARMD can be followed with home Amsler, and repeat DFE in
      6 – 12 months depending on severity
   3) Counsel patients that smoking, hypertension, and sun exposure
      are risk factors
   4) Zinc and antioxidant vitamins have been proven to have a small
      but significant benefit in slowing the progression of ARMD
   5) A diet rich in lutein and zeaxanthin appears to be even more
      beneficial, though less well proven so far. Recommended foods
      include kale, collard greens, and spinach, and to a lesser extent,
      broccoli, brussels sprouts, leaf lettuce, green peas and summer
      squash
   6) Many supplements containing lutein are now available. The
      recommended minimum dose is 6 mg po
   7) Omega 3 in cold-water fish also appears to slow progression
      about 30%. Recommend 3 servings of tuna, salmon, or sardines
      per week, or 1000 mg fish oil capsules tid with meals
   8) 6 – 40 mg of lutein, 40 mg of zinc, and antioxidants with 3000 mg
      of fish oil is probably the best recommendation until definitive
      studies are reported

Notes____

____

____

____

____

____

____

11

DIABETES

A) Subjective
1) Half of all diabetics may be undiagnosed. Incidence is increasing with population aging and increased obesity. Diabetic retinopathy is the leading cause of blindness in the US, ages 20 – 65
   Symptoms include
   a) Increased thirst
   b) Hunger
   c) Urination
   d) Tiredness
   e) Unplanned weight loss
   f) Blurred vision
   g) Paresthesia
   h) Frequent infection
   i) Slow healing wounds
   j) Impotence
2) Vision may or may not be affected yet. 50% have retinopathy after 7 yrs
3) Diabetes that can be controlled by diet is less likely to cause retinopathy
4) Type 1 diabetes (juvenile) is more likely than Type 2 (adult onset) to cause retinopathy
5) Insulin controlled is more likely than oral controlled to cause retinopathy. Insulin types
   a) R: Regular, short acting (3 – 6 hrs) (Humulin R, Novolin R)
   b) S: Semilente, short acting
   c) N: NPH, intermediate onset and duration of effect (10 – 20 hrs) (Humulin 70/30, Novolin 70/30)
   d) L: Lente, intermediate onset and duration of effect
   e) U: Ultralente, long acting (20 – 36 hrs) (Humulin U)
   f) 50/50: 50% NPH and 50% regular combination
   g) 70/30: 70% NPH and 30% regular combination
6) Oral diabetic medications
   a) Second generation sulfonylureas: glipizide (Glucotrol), glyburide (DiaBeta, Micronase, Glynase), glimepiride (Amaryl)
      1) Stimulate insulin secretion, increase insulin sensitivity, decrease glucose output

          2) Common side effects: hypoglycemia, rash, photophobia, GI upset, weight gain

       b) Meglitinides: repaglinide (Prandin), nateglinide (Starlix)

          1) Stimulate insulin secretion rapidly

          2) Common side effects: hypoglycemia, weight gain

       c) Biguanides: metformin (Glucophage)

          1) Decrease glucose output and increase uptake

          2) No hypoglycemia, reduced weight gain, decrease triglycerides but can cause anorexia and nausea. Dangerous with alcohol and iodinated materials such as CT contrast dye

       d) Alpha-glucosidase inhibitors: acarbose (Precose), miglitol (Glyset)

          1) Inhibits alpha-glucosidase, decrease post-prandial hyperglycemia (*i.e.*, reduce carbohydrate digestion after meals)

          2) Common side effects: GI disturbance

       e) Thiazolidinedione (TZD): rosiglitazone (Avandia), pioglitazone (Actos)

          1) Promotes glucose uptake by making cells more sensitive to natural insulin

          2) Common side effects: hepatotoxicity, edema, anemia, weight gain

       f) Combination drugs

          1) Metformin/glyburide (Glucovance)

          2) Rosiglitazone/metformin (Advandamet)

7) Morning blood glucose readings above 155 mg/dL or unstable readings are more likely to cause early retinopathy

8) Glycosylated hemoglobin (HbA1c) readings above 7.2% are more likely to cause early retinopathy. HbA1c measures average blood glucose level over the last 8 – 12 weeks and is a better indication of compliance and control than blood glucose levels

9) Hypertension, hypercholesterolemia and other cardiovascular diseases are risk factors for retinopathy

10) Goals

       a) Glucose before meal 80 – 120

       b) Glucose after meal 100 – 140

       c) HbA1c (glycosylated hemoglobin) <7%

HbA1c table

		Needs Improvement						Good		Very Good		
HbA1c test score		14.0	13.0	12.0	11.0	10.0	9.0	8.0	7.0	6.0	5.0	4.0
Mean Blood Glucose	mg/dL	380	350	315	280	250	215	180	150	115	80	50
	mmol/L	21.1	19.3	17.4	15.6	13.7	11.9	10.0	8.2	6.3	4.7	2.6

B) Objective

1) VA and pinhole or best corrected VA (watch for refractive changes)
2) BP
3) Pupils
4) Extraocular eye movements to R/O diabetic palsies
5) Cover test or von Graefe phorias to document baseline phoria. Later, if diplopia occurs, a high pre-existing phoria may indicate a decompensating phoria instead of a diabetic palsy
6) External and slit lamp exam
    a) Look for diabetic corneal striae, reduced sensitivity and abrasions
    b) R/O rubeosis (neovascularization of the iris) (NVI)
    c) R/O diabetic cataracts or any other opacity that may be reducing visual acuity (initially appear as snow-white opacities within cortex or posterior capsule)
    d) Poor pupil dilation
7) Dilated fundus examination with BIO, 90 D and, if necessary, a fundus contact lens
    a) Note any dot or blot hemorrhages and cotton wool spots (NPDR) (previously known as BDR)
    b) Look for venous beading and loops
    c) Look for intraretinal microvascular abnormalities (IRMA)
    d) R/O neovascularization of the disk (NVD) or elsewhere (NVE)
    e) Look for any hard exudates in the macular area indicating a chronic serous leakage
    f) Look for any microaneurysms or blot hemorrhages at or around the macula
    g) Using your stereopsis and a fundus contact lens if necessary, R/O any retinal thickening in the macular area. Look carefully around any hard exudates
8) Monocular color vision testing, preferably with Farnsworth D-15; a blue-yellow loss may indicate early macular damage if clear media

C) Assessment: does this patient need fluorescein angiography or laser treatment? Early treatment of diabetes retinopathy study (ETDRS) guidelines

1) Non-proliferative diabetic retinopathy (NPDR)
    a) Mild NPDR or background diabetic retinopathy (BDR)
        1) At least 1 dot microaneurysm
    b) Moderate NPDR or BDR, any **1** of the following
        1) Hemorrhages and/or microaneurysms greater than that shown in ETDRS Standard Photo 2A (see Figure 11-1 on pg. 77) in any 1 quadrant
            a) Dot microaneurysms and blot hemorrhages located in outer plexiform and inner nuclear layers
            b) Flame hemorrhage located in nerve fiber layer
        2) Soft exudates (cotton wool spots)

           3) Venous beading in 1 quadrant
           4) Intraretinal microvascular abnormalities (IRMA)
       c) Severe NPDR, any 1 of the following
           1) Hemorrhage or microaneurysms greater than ETDRS standard photo 2A (see Figure 11-1 on pg. 77) in all 4 quadrants
           2) Venous beading in 2 quadrants
           3) Intraretinal vascular abnormalities greater than ETDRS standard photo 8A in 1 quadrant (see Figure 11-2 on pg. 77)
       d) Very severe NPDR
           1) 2 or more lesions of severe NPDR
    2) Early proliferative diabetic retinopathy (PDR)
       a) Neovascularization is present but it does not meet the high risk definition
       b) Any PDR warrants a FANG and a retina consultation
    3) High risk PDR, (neovascularization) requiring treatment
       a) NVD greater than ¼ – ⅓ disk diameter in size; see ETDRS standard photo 10A (see Figure 11-3 on pg. 77)
       b) Any NVD with preretinal or vitreous heme
       c) NVE greater than ½ disk diameter in size with a preretinal or vitreous heme
       d) Any NVI
    4) Clinically significant diabetic macular edema definition (CSDME)
       a) Any retinal edema or thickening within ⅓ disk diameter of the fovea
       b) Any hard exudates within ⅓ disk diameter of the center of the macula with any adjacent edema, even if that edema is more than ⅓ disk diameter away from the fovea
       c) An area of retinal edema greater than 1 disk diameter in size, if any part of the edema is within 1 disk diameter of the fovea
       d) Note: any marginal macular edema as seen ophthalmoscopically should have a fluorescein angiography done for definitive classification
    5) Diabetic eye disease should be bilateral. If there is a significant difference between the eyes, consider
       a) Carotid insufficiency on side of better eye, protecting it from hypertensive damage. Listen for bruit and/or medical referral
       b) Branch or central vein occlusion: more hemorrhages with adjacent narrowing of arterioles

D) Plan
    1) No retinopathy
       a) Counsel about importance of strict blood glucose control, exercise, BP control, and weight loss to delay onset of retinopathy. Lipid and hypertension control will help reduce the incidence of diabetic macular edema
       b) RTC in 1 yr for DFE
       c) Send report to physician

2) Mild NPDR
   a) Counsel 15% incidence of high risk retinopathy in 5 yrs and remind of the need for strict glucose control, exercise, BP control, and weight loss to delay worsening of retinopathy. Lipid and hypertension control will help reduce the incidence of diabetic macular edema
   b) RTC in 1 yr for DFE
   c) Send report to physician
3) Moderate NPDR
   a) Counsel 27% incidence of high risk retinopathy in 5 yrs and remind of the need for strict glucose control, exercise, BP control, and weight loss to delay worsening of retinopathy. Lipid and hypertension control will help reduce the incidence of diabetic macular edema
   b) RTC in 4 months for DFE
   c) Send report to physician
4) Severe or very severe NPDR (pre-proliferative)
   a) Counsel 15% incidence of high risk retinopathy in 1 yr and 56% in 5 yrs. Remind of the need for strict glucose control, exercise, BP control, and weight loss to limit worsening of retinopathy. Lipid and hypertension control will help reduce the incidence of diabetic macular edema
   b) RTC in 2 – 3 months and consider fluorescein angiography or retina consult
   c) Send report to physician
5) Early PDR (may have proliferative disease with little NPDR)
   a) Counsel that high risk retinopathy is present and strict glucose control is necessary; though a sudden tightening of glucose control may cause a temporary worsening of retinopathy, it is still better in the long term
   b) Order fluorescein angiography or retina consult for possible early panretinal photocoagulation (PRP). Warn that PRP may cause a temporary reduction of vision
   c) Send report to physician
6) High risk PDR
   a) Order a retina consult for PRP within 48 hrs
   b) Send report to physician
7) During pregnancy
   a) Monitor each trimester
   b) Send report to physician
8) Diabetic macular edema **not** meeting CSDME criteria with unaffected VA
   a) Counsel need for strict glucose control, exercise, BP control and weight loss to delay onset of retinopathy. Lipid and hypertension control will help reduce the incidence of diabetic macular edema
   b) Monitor every 3 months with DFE and do home Amsler Grid
   c) Consider fluorescein angiography or retina consult, especially if the fellow eye had a difficult course with macular edema

       d) Send report to physician

9) CSDME or reduced VA
   a) Counsel need for strict glucose control, exercise, BP control and weight loss to delay onset of retinopathy. Lipid and hypertension control will help the diabetic macular edema
   b) Refer for retina consult and focal grid laser or intravitreal Kenalog injection
   c) Send report to physician

10) NVI
   a) Counsel risk of imminent vision loss
   b) Refer for retina consult and PRP, STAT
   c) Send report to physician

11) Vitreous hemorrhage
   a) Call physician and get approval to discontinue any aspirin or blood thinner prescribed
   b) Refer for retina consult, B-scan ultrasound, PRP or vitrectomy ASAP

12) There is a high mortality rate of patients with diabetic retinopathy; 61% of original ETDRS patients died within 13 – 19.5 yrs. Of the survivors, 42% had 20/20 or better, 84% had 20/40 or better. 20% lost 3 or more lines of vision from baseline

13) BP control reduces the risk of diabetic retinopathy by 50%

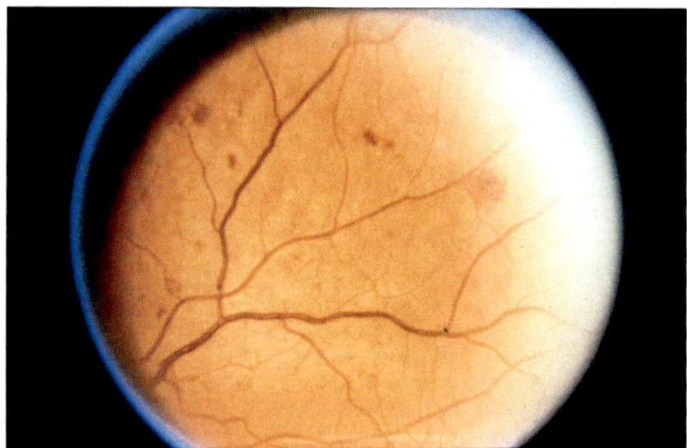

Figure 11-1

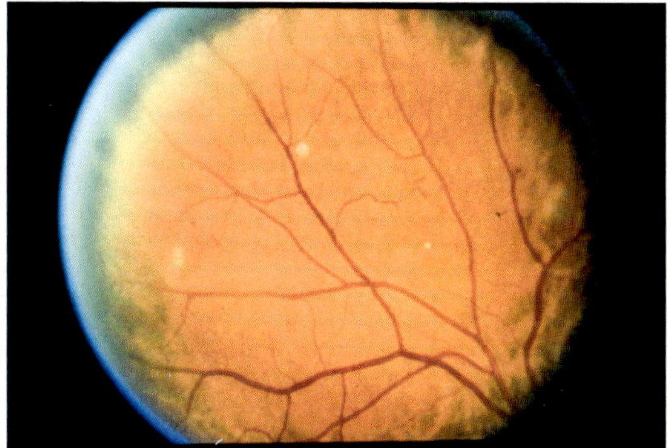

Figure 11-2

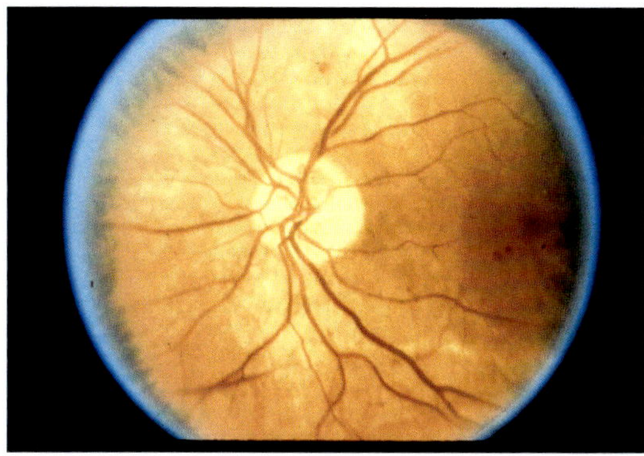

Figure 11-3

Notes

12

HYPERTENSIVE RETINOPATHY

A) Subjective
1) Usually no complaints
2) A history of high BP is often known

B) Objective
1) VA and pinhole or best corrected VA
2) Extraocular eye movement testing
3) Cover testing or von Graefe phorias to document any phoria that may later decompensate
4) Pupil testing
5) Measure BP
6) External and slit lamp: R/O subconjunctival hemorrhage
7) DFE: expect bilateral presentation, look for the following in increasing order of seriousness
   a) Narrowing of arterioles
   b) Arteriole/venous crossing defects
   c) Widening of the arteriole light reflex causing a silver or copper wire appearance
   d) Cotton wool spots
   e) Hard exudates
   f) Retinal hemorrhage (especially flame hemorrhage) or microaneurysms
   g) Optic nerve swelling
8) Blood glucose measurement

C) Assessment/Plan: either systolic or diastolic over these limits counts in evaluation
1) <120 systolic or <80 diastolic: normal, recheck in 2 yrs
2) 120 – 139 systolic or 80 – 89 diastolic: prehypertension, recheck in 1 yr and make lifestyle changes
3) 140 – 159 systolic or 90 – 99 diastolic: stage I hypertension, have medical doctor confirm within 2 months
4) 160 – 179 systolic or 100 – 109 diastolic: stage II hypertension, have medical doctor evaluate in 1 month
5) 180 systolic or 110 diastolic without clinical symptoms requires medical intervention within 1 week

    6) 180 systolic or 110 diastolic with any of the following is a medical emergency; refer to the emergency department if the family physician is not immediately available. Examples include
        a) Hemorrhage of the conjunctiva, vitreous, or retina: family physician OK
        b) Headache: family physician OK
        c) Optic nerve swelling: send to emergency department
        d) Sudden blurred vision: send to emergency department
        e) Chest pain: call ambulance for emergency department
        f) Difficulty breathing: call ambulance for emergency department
    7) Ocular signs should be bilateral. If unilateral consider the following
        a) Carotid insufficiency on side of better eye, protecting it from hypertensive damage. Listen for bruit and/or medical doctor referral
        b) Branch or central vein occlusion (more hemorrhages with no arteriole narrowing)
    8) BP control cuts risk of diabetic retinopathy by 50% in diabetics

D) Follow up
    1) Primary treatment is by the family physician
    2) Follow ocular changes in 2 – 12 months, depending on severity

Notes ____

____

____

____

____

____

____

____

____

____

____

____

____

____

13

PERIPHERAL RETINA (FLASHES AND FLOATERS)

A) Subjective: retinal breaks must be ruled out if any 1 of the following Sx are present
   1) Any monocular flashing light in peripheral vision not accompanied by classic migraine Sx
   2) Any new onset of floaters or shadow in vision
   3) Any sudden loss of vision

B) Objective
   1) VA and pinhole or best corrected VA
   2) Pupils: afferent pupillary defect is possible if large detachment is present
   3) Confrontation visual fields: important! A large, shallow detachment may be hard to find ophthalmoscopically but poor fields will be evident with confrontation visual fields
   4) Slit lamp: look for pigment in the vitreous (Schaffer's sign)
   5) IOP: monocular low IOP is likely to be retinal detachment (RD)
   6) Get full dilation: use 10% phenylephrine if necessary
   7) DFE: scleral depression
      a) Use a 28 or 30 D lens for a larger field of view. A +8 D cap on a +20 D lens has a larger diameter than a dedicated +28 or +30 lens
      b) Use a good Storz E-5108 stainless steel depressor for control and ease of use
      c) Recline patient if possible, look carefully
      d) Instill a topical anesthetic
      e) Depress area of the retina corresponding to the flashes, at a minimum. You should attempt a 360° depression on all flashes and floaters. Young tight lids might make this very difficult
      f) Do not hesitate to depress sclera directly at 3 and 9 if lids are too tight. Clean depressor and use topical anesthetic
      g) Look for red holes
      h) Look for an operculum floating in vitreous
      i) Some flaps cannot be seen unless depressed!
      j) Do not be fooled by a prominent vitreous base
      k) Large, low lying detachments can be hard to see; look for a loss of choroidal detail

l) Try to find the hole (many have multiple holes). The hole is usually at the top edge of the detached area and can be very small

m) In pseudophakia, the hole is likely to be superior, or near the surgical wound

8) DFE: 3-mirror examination — do on all high risk patients to find small holes and tears

C) Assessment
1) High risk findings
- a) Retinal detachment
    1) If a detachment line is walled off with pigment and no Sx, no emergency. Refer, since many will eventually progress
    2) If the macula is on, or partly on, STAT referral
    3) If the macula is already completely off with hand motion vision, up to a 1 week delay will not make a difference
- b) Retinal hole
    1) If you find a hole without pigment with Sx, refer for focal and/or pneumatic retinopexy urgently
    2) An inferior, non-pigmented hole probably should be observed closely if there are no flashes or floaters, but should have focal laser treatment if Sx are present (talk to your retina specialist; they differ in their management)
- c) Flap or horseshoe tears
    1) Some flap tears may not be visible until depressed!
    2) Urgent retina referral, traction may still be present
- d) Operculated holes
    1) The operculum may be more visible in the vitreous with BIO than the hole itself
    2) If not old and pigmented, refer
2) Lower risk findings
- a) Prominent vitreous base
    1) Pale wide bands of silky white in the periphery
    2) Due to vitreous-retina interface abnormality
    3) Can be confused with a detachment
        a) R/O any holes and opercula, especially at the superior part of the white area
        b) Use scleral depression to R/O flap tears and low lying detachments
        c) Choroidal detail should still be visible through the white area if it is attached (a fresh detachment will be edematous and obscure the view of the choroid)
    4) More common in blacks
    5) Benign, though a subsequent vitreous detachment is more likely to result in a tear here due to a stronger attachment
- b) Cobblestone or paving stone degeneration
    1) Large round, yellow lesions, usually with surrounding pigment
    2) R/O any fluid cuff or retinal elevation indicating a true hole

      3) Benign
  c) Cystic tufts
      1) Retinal thickening and cysts
      2) Mild risk of tear
  d) Lattice degeneration
      1) Long, narrow areas of degeneration running parallel to equator
      2) May have associated atrophic holes without cuff of detachment
         a) A true hole can be distinguished from thinning only with scleral indentation or 3-mirror inspection
      3) A 2 – 4% risk of a future retinal detachment
      4) Counsel, and consider prophylactic laser if high risk, such as pseudophakia, high myopia, or previous history of detachment
  e) Retinoschisis
      1) Due to a splitting between retinal layers
      2) Must be differentiated from a retinal detachment
         a) Retinoschisis usually does not have holes. When a break in the inner (close to vitreous) layer is present, a retina consult is advised to be safe. A break in the outer layer could allow retinal detachment and is more dangerous
         b) The surface is smooth, transparent and rigid with eye movement, not loose, milky, and undulating with eye movement, such as in a retinal detachment
         c) Depression pushes the elevated area away from the depressor. A detached area will deflate because the associated hole allows fluid under the detachment to escape
         d) Schisis causes absolute field loss due to separation of the retinal layers. Detachment causes a relative field loss because although the retina is sick, the connections to the optic nerve are intact
         e) Schisis is not associated with a sudden onset of flashes and floaters
  f) Reticular degeneration
      1) Pigmented honeycomb-like pattern in the periphery
      2) Usually in the elderly
      3) Benign
  g) Congenital hypertrophy of the retinal pigment epithelium (CHRPE, Bear Tracks)
      1) Very dark margins
      2) May be only a dark ring
      3) Benign
      4) If present 360° and bilateral, Gardner's familial polyposis. High risk of colon cancer. Refer for colonoscopy
  h) Nevus
      1) Flat, yellow drusen may be present

  i) Melanoma
    1) Elevated, orange pigment may be present

D) Plan
1) If urgent referral is indicated, phone your retina consultant and arrange the appointment to ensure follow up
2) If flashes and/or floaters are present and the retina is OK, diagnose vitreous traction or vitreous detachment depending on presence of a posterior vitreous detachment (PVD)
3) Document warning the patient to return immediately if flashes or floaters worsen significantly or he/she sees a veil or note a loss of vision
4) RTC in 3 weeks all newly symptomatic patients not needing referral

E) Follow up
1) Repeat the entire exam
2) Statistically, most retinal defects in symptomatic patients will show up in the first 3 weeks
3) If symptoms are still pronounced at 3 weeks, RTC again

Notes

14

SUDDEN MONOCULAR VISION LOSS
WITH RETINAL CHANGES

A) Central retinal artery occlusion (CRAO)
1) Subjective: sudden painless monocular vision loss
2) Objective
    a) Cherry red spot in the macula
    b) Pale edematous retina
3) Assessment: did it occur less than 6 hrs ago?
4) Plan
    a) If <6 hrs onset
        1) Have the patient breathe in bag
        2) Do 10 sec globe compression with a 3-mirror until pulsation of retinal arteries followed by 5 sec release for up to 20 min (monitor pulse for bradycardia)
        3) Instill 1 of each category of glaucoma drops
        4) Oral glycerol (or isosorbide if diabetic) per instructions
        5) Call your retina specialist to do paracentesis to lower the IOP if no improvement after 20 min. Also may use other systemic treatment to improve circulation
    b) Do BP, blood glucose and temporal arteritis workup STAT including history and labs (see Chapter 15)
    c) Evaluate the fellow eye
    d) Refer for systemic evaluation of heart, carotids, blood dyscrasias and for retina consult

B) Central retinal vein occlusion (CRVO)
1) Subjective: sudden painless monocular vision loss
2) Objective
    a) Retinal hemorrhages in all 4 quadrants
    b) Cotton wool spots may be visible
    c) Dilated, tortuous, retinal veins
3) Assessment: 2 types
    a) Perfused or venous stasis: less hemorrhage, VA 20/400 or better, ⅓ improve, ⅓ stable, ⅓ worsen
    b) Non-perfused or ischemic: less than 20/400, more hemorrhage, 50 – 80% develop neovascularization of the iris in 3 months unless pan retinal photocoagulation

       c) 10% become bilateral or go from perfused to ischemic
    4) Plan
       a) Do BP and blood glucose in office
       b) Start aspirin 1 tab po qd
       c) Refer for systemic evaluation soon (R/O hypertension and diabetes)
         1) If bilateral R/O hyperviscosity
         2) If mostly peripheral hemorrhage R/O carotid insufficiency
       d) Get a retina consult. They will watch every 2 – 3 weeks for NVI and for hemorrhage to clear, then do FANG

C) Branch retinal vein occlusion (BRVO)

    1) Subjective: symptoms vary
       a) Sudden, monocular painless loss of central vision
       b) Sudden, monocular painless loss of peripheral vision
       c) Asymptomatic
    2) Objective
       a) Heme and retinal edema in a wedge shaped pattern starting at an arteriole venous crossing
       b) Macular edema may be present depending on location
    3) Assessment
       a) Is enough blood present to block a view of fluorescein?
       b) Is initial VA <20/100? Indicates fovea ischemia, worse outcome
    4) Plan
       a) Do gonioscopy and slit lamp for iris neovascularization
       b) Do BP and blood glucose in your office
       c) Order a systemic evaluation
       d) Start 1 aspirin tab po qd
       e) RTC in 1 month. No need to refer yet unless edema is threatening the macula
       f) Repeat gonioscopy at each visit (for NVI)
       g) After the blood mostly clears in 3 – 6 months refer for FANG and focal laser
         1) Laser treatment will be used if VA <20/40 due to chronic macular edema
         2) Panretinal photocoagulation (PRP) for neovascularization; early treatment is no help. Laser reduces all risk 50%
         3) After laser RTC in 3 – 4 months; if improving RTC in 3 – 4 months, if not improving repeat FANG
         4) Always perform gonioscopy carefully for neovascularization of the iris

D) Central serous maculopathy

    1) Subjective: sudden, painless monocular vision loss or distortion (mild to moderate)
       a) Mild to moderate blur or distortion, not as bad as in choroidal neovascular membrane (CNVM)
       b) Classically, males 23 – 50, monocular

        c) Usually have identifiable high stress factor
        d) Half of patients with central serous in one study had used systemic steroids in the past month or had Cushing's disease
    2) Objective
        a) Characteristic serous dome covering the fovea
        b) Be sure to get a good binocular view, there are few monocular cues, the dome merges gradually with normal retina
        c) Use a fundus contact lens if in doubt
        d) Distortion of Amsler, a relative scotoma, not absolute
    3) Assessment
        a) R/O other macular disease
        b) FANG, if >age 60 or chorio retinal scars
    4) Plan
        a) Counsel, discontinue systemic steroids if possible. R/O Cushing's disease. RTC in 6 weeks
        b) If not resolved in 2 – 3 months, do FANG
        c) Resolution will leave some RPE disruption and perhaps mild vision and contrast sensitivity loss. Just be sure the retina is flat and dry

E) Choroidal neovascular membrane (CNVM)
    1) Subjective: sudden painless monocular vision loss, distortion or scotoma in elderly
    2) Objective
        a) More pronounced VA loss and Amsler changes
        b) Usually (but not always) preexisting ARMD, histoplasmosis, or other retinal disease
        c) Have more monocular clues than central serous, often subretinal heme, pigment, dirty gray-green color and exudates
        d) May be subtle or completely occult; use a fundus contact lens if necessary
    3) Assessment: any new central vision change on Amsler except central serous needs FANG within 24 hrs
    4) Plan: refer to a retina specialist for FANG and possible laser STAT

F) Macular hole
    1) Subjective: sudden, painless, monocular loss of vision
    2) Objective: use a fundus contact lens and a good slit lamp
    3) Assessment: have patient look at middle of a thin slit. If distortion or gap in beam is noted, diagnose macular hole vs. a pseudo hole in an epiretinal membrane (Watzke Allen test)
        a) Impending
            1) Mild to moderate vision loss
            2) Small elevation or loss of pit in fovea, yellow spot or ring is visible: stage 1
            3) May have a small tear at the edge of the spot: stage 2
        b) Full thickness macular hole
            1) 20/200 VA

        2) Small red hole in fovea with surrounding cuff of subsensory fluid and intracellular edema
        3) An epiretinal membrane is usually visible
        4) If no posterior vitreous detachment is present: stage 3
        5) If a PVD is present: stage 4
    4) Plan
        a) Stage 1 impending hole: monitor closely with Amsler grid and follow up dilated exams
        b) Stage 2 impending hole: STAT retina consult for vitrectomy to relieve circumferential traction caused by the epiretinal membrane; usually done if VA <20/40
        c) Stage 3 or 4 (hole): order a non-urgent retina consult. Pars plana vitrectomy (PPV) with membrane peel (MP), gas bubble and face down positioning often give dramatic resolution
        d) The second eye is at a high risk. Close follow up with Amsler grid is necessary. Surgery is done at the first Sx in the second eye

G) Vitreous hemorrhage
    1) Subjective
        a) Sudden painless monocular vision loss, onset of floaters or webs
        b) Hx: usually a reason such as diabetes, retinal tear or vitreous detachment
    2) Objective
        a) Look carefully with BIO and 28 or 30 D lens with scleral depression
        b) Look at the other eye for clues to the etiology (diabetes, high myopia, etc.)
        c) If the view is too poor, order a B-scan
    3) Assessment: retinal tears, holes and detachments must be ruled out
    4) Plan
        a) Enforced bed rest with 45° elevation
        b) No reading (too many saccades), TV OK
        c) No aspirin, NSAID, or other anticoagulants
        d) Retina consult in 2 days

Notes ____

____

____

____

____

____

15

NEUROVASCULAR SUDDEN VISION LOSS
(NO OPHTHALMOSCOPIC CAUSE FOUND)

A) Subjective
1) Sudden monocular vision loss
2) Ask if pain on eye movement, paresthesia or weakness due to heat or other Sx

B) Objective
1) VA and pinhole or best corrected VA
2) Pupils: look for APD or other pupil defects
3) Extra ocular eye movements: R/O 3rd nerve palsy
4) Confrontation visual fields: carefully note any defects. Minor losses may be missed with confrontation. Do 30° threshold or Goldmann fields
5) Monocular color vision testing: red cap test or the best color vision test you have in the office, done monocularly
6) External/exophthalmometry: R/O proptosis
7) Slit lamp: R/O hyphema and other abnormalities
8) DFE: R/O vitreous hemorrhage, artery and vein occlusions and macular abnormalities. Look for edema or hemorrhage of the optic nerve
9) Check BP
10) Check random blood glucose in office

C) Assessment: sudden, painless, monocular vision loss caused by vascular problems are suspected after you have excluded all ocular causes
1) Giant cell arteritis or temporal arteritis (GCA)
   a) Assessment
      1) A true vision-threatening emergency. If you can start tests before the internist sees the patient, you will save time and morbidity
      2) Must be ruled out in all elderly patients (>55, but especially >75) with sudden vision loss. The loss may be central (Snellen) or peripheral (confrontation fields)
      3) Risk factors
         a) Jaw claudication = 9x risk!

            b) Neck or occipital pain = 3.4x risk

            c) >75 yrs old = 2x risk

            d) Temple or scalp tenderness is not predictive!

            e) C-reactive protein >2.45 mg/dL = 3.2x risk. 100% sensitive

            f) Sed rate >47 = 2x risk. Sed rate >107 = 2.7x risk (5 – 10% of temporal arteritis patients have normal sed rates!)

            g) A positive C-reactive protein >2.45 mg/dL combined with sed rate >47 is 97% specific

            h) Platelets >400 mm³ are a marker for temporal arteritis

            i) White race is a risk factor. Temporal arteritis occurs rarely in Hispanics and blacks

            j) Polymyalgia rheumatica (moderate to severe muscle pain and stiffness in the neck, shoulders and hips, most often in women >50): 15% incidence in giant cell

       4) With sudden, monocular vision loss when the patient is >55 (but especially if >75) you must ask about a history of

            a) Jaw claudication

            b) Neck or occipital pain

            c) Scalp tenderness

            d) A tender scalp or temples, with anorexia or weight loss are classic symptoms that should cause you to order the lab tests, but these Sx do not help predict which patients will have a positive biopsy

       5) A painful temple may also indicate herpes zoster (shingles). Look for vesicles, monitor closely or refer to internist while watching for ocular involvement

D) Plan: common sense advice but no easy answers

       1) If the Sx are strong (*e.g.*, elderly patient, sudden unexplained vision loss, jaw claudication or other related Sx), send to an internist (get labs started first to save time) or emergency department (can do labs there)

            a) Order a STAT sed rate, C-reactive protein, CBC with differential

            b) Use the sed rate (results take 2 hrs) and the above Sx to decide if referral and biopsy are needed

                1) Strong Sx with a high sed rate confirms

                     a) STAT referral for oral steroids and a temporal artery biopsy

                     b) Oral steroids should be started while arranging the biopsy

                     c) The biopsy will have to be done within 2 weeks of starting steroids, or the steroids will affect it

                2) Strong Sx with normal sed rate means nothing; biopsy

                3) The C-reactive protein is very useful. It should be ready when the sed rate is done, but some labs have to send it out so results can take longer

        4) Platelets >400 mm³ are less sensitive but more specific for temporal arteritis than the sed rate

2) If the Sx (*i.e.*, the above temporal arteritis hallmark Sx) are weak or absent in a patient >age 55 with sudden vision loss, temporal arteritis must be ruled out with a history and lab work (CBC, STAT sed rate and C-reactive protein) if no other explanation is found. Wait for the C-reactive protein results

  a) If the sed rate is high: refer

    1) Weak Sx and a sed >107: 95% chance of temporal arteritis or malignancy, infection, or other collagen vascular disorder; refer to an internist

    2) Weak Sx and a sed between 48 and 107: grey zone, refer for biopsy or empiric steroid trial while waiting for C-reactive test and platelet count

  b) If the sed rate is normal

    1) Weak Sx and normal sed rate <1%: chance of temporal arteritis

    2) 22% of temporal arteritis patients have a normal sed rate, but they probably have Sx, or a high C-reactive protein, or high platelet count. They may also have a high sed rate on another day

    3) Look at the C-reactive and platelet results

      a) If either is high, refer

      b) If both are normal and the central and peripheral vision is consistent with known ocular pathology: monitor closely with acuities, pupils, monocular color and 30-2 fields

      c) If both are normal and the vision is acutely reduced, it is probably nonarteritic anterior ischemic optic neuropathy or an occult retinal problem. Consider referral to a neuro and/or retina ophthalmologist

3) Non-arteritic anterior ischemic optic neuropathy (NAION)

  a) Assessment

    1) Younger ages: 40 and up

    2) Sudden painless loss, often on awakening (nocturnal hypotension)

    3) Hx of vascular disease (HTN, diabetes, atherosclerosis, stroke, carotid occlusion)

    4) Also a crowded disk, GI ulcers or other blood loss, or migraine Hx may be contributory

    5) Altitudinal VF loss

    6) Disk swelling may be present early, often segmental, flame hemorrhages; pallor appears later

    7) You must R/O temporal arteritis by history and labs (see above)

  b) Plan

    1) Start 1 aspirin per day and have patient seen by medical doctor soon; medical doctor may consider stopping p.m. BP meds (controversial)

2) Spontaneous partial improvement in 42%
3) 30% progress within 6 months
4) 7% progress in 6 weeks
5) 40% become bilateral in 2 yrs
6) Monitor 1 – 2 weeks

4) Papilledema vs. crowded nerve head
   a) Assessment
      1) Papilledema and the underlying increased intracranial pressure may be asymptomatic in mild cases
      2) Intermittent bilateral visual loss or diplopia associated with posture changes may occur with papilledema
      3) Tinnitus may occur
      4) Increased intracranial pressure may cause
         a) Severe headaches, throbbing, non-localized, episodic, worse in the morning
         b) Nausea, usually associated with headaches
         c) Stiff neck: ask the patient to bend neck until chin touches chest. Pain indicates inflamed meninges, usually due to cranial infection
      5) DFE: papilledema signs
         a) Blurring of disk margins
         b) Disk hemorrhages
         c) Swelling of the nerve fiber layer: obscures underlying vessels
         d) Congested, pink nerve head
         e) Venous stasis
      6) DFE: buried drusen signs
         a) Pale, yellow color to nerve head
         b) Irregular scalloped edge to elevated area
         c) Transilluminate 1 edge of the elevated areas with a slit beam. The entire elevation will glow if buried drusen are present
      7) DFE: hypoplastic optic nerve signs
         a) Select the middle size spot in the new Welch Allyn ophthalmoscope with 3 sizes, or the small spot in the older heads with 2 spots. With a Keeler direct, use the outer bull's eye ring
         b) The normal nerve head is the same size as this spot when projected in the eye
         c) A nerve head that is significantly smaller than this spot is hypoplastic and may not have papilledema
         d) Hypoplasia does not cause blurring of disk margins
   b) Plan
      1) Refer to neurologist for an MRI and possible lumbar puncture with measurement of opening pressures if you suspect true papilledema
         a) Pseudotumor cerebri: idiopathic intracranial hypertension is a diagnosis of exclusion
            1) Criteria

    a) Signs and symptoms of increased intracranial pressure
    b) An awake and alert patient
    c) No localized neurologic signs (except VI paresis)
    d) Increased CSF pressure but no other abnormalities
    e) Normal-to-small symmetrical ventricles with neuro-imaging
   2) Untreated, it can cause permanent peripheral vision loss, similar to glaucoma
   3) Often in obese young females
   4) Treated by weight loss of 6%. Diamox and occasionally the surgical placement of a shunt may also be used. The weight loss is vital
  b) Space occupying lesions of the head: neurosurgical referral
 5) Optic neuritis (inflammation)
  a) Assessment
   1) Sudden, rapid progression of vision loss. May be worsened by increased body temperature after the neuritis is healed
   2) Unilateral
   3) More likely in young females
   4) Pain on palpation or eye movement
   5) Variable VA loss, up to 20/200 or worse, though may be better in early stages
   6) Variable field loss, usually in the central 30°
   7) Positive red cap test or monocular color vision difference if the VA is affected
   8) Exophthalmometry results normal
   9) Papillitis (unilateral findings)
    a) Blurred disk margins and other papilledema signs
    b) Findings are unilateral (as opposed to bilateral papilledema)
    c) White blood cells in the vitreous may form a haze
   10) Retrobulbar neuritis
    a) All of the above Sx with a normal nerve head because the inflammation is located further back in the optic nerve
  b) Plan
   1) Order an MRI with thin sections through the orbits and brain to look for peri-ventricular demyelinating plaques (multiple sclerosis)
   2) Refer to a neurologist. Viral and granulomatous diseases will have to be ruled out if no MS is found
   3) Early intervention in optic neuritis with IV steroids will cause faster VA recovery and the rate of developing MS (if several plaques are found on MRI) is cut from 36% to 16% for 2 yrs. There is no benefit thereafter

        4) Weekly Avonex injections greatly reduce the progression of lesions on MRI

        5) The long term prognosis for MS is better when optic neuritis is the initial presentation than when other symptoms occur first

6) Amaurosis fugax
   a) Assessment
      1) It is transient! Lasts for seconds up to 24 hrs. You can R/O a lot of bad things already
      2) Listen to carotids and take BP
      3) Look for Hollenhorst plaques
      4) Look at systemic history and age. Take a giant cell arteritis Hx if 55 or older
   b) Plan: refer to an internist

7) Classic migraine: all of the above are negative and a non-elderly patient
   a) Assessment
      1) Vision loss is followed by a bad headache
      2) Scintillating auras, often colored lights
      3) Monocular or binocular
      4) Nausea or vague feeling of illness or mental impairment
      5) Photophobia
      6) Possible Hx of birth control pills or Premarin
   b) Plan: counsel or refer to family doctor

8) Ocular migraine: visual aura without the headache, a diagnosis of exclusion

Notes ____

____

____

____

____

____

____

____

____

____

____

____

16

OCULOMOTOR PROBLEMS (DIPLOPIA AND PTOSIS)

A) Subjective
1) Vary, but include central or peripheral vision loss with or without pain, sudden diplopia, sudden ptosis and pupil abnormalities

B) Objective
1) VA and pinhole or best corrected VA
2) Pupils: use a bright light and look carefully for
    a) Anisocoria
    b) Direct pupil response
    c) Consensual response
    d) Afferent pupil defect or reverse afferent pupil defect
    e) Near response
3) Eye movements
4) Cover test: with 3-step test for diplopia (see assessment)
5) External: R/O exophthalmos, measure ptosis if present
6) Use a Hertel ophthalmometer on all potential orbital problems
7) Red cap test or monocular color vision testing for all cases of optic nerve problems or monocular vision loss without an ocular cause
8) Confrontation visual fields on all patients, threshold (30°) or Goldmann fields when indicated
9) Slit lamp
10) DFE
    a) BIO with scleral depression, if necessary, to R/O retinal detachments
    b) Fundus lens evaluation of disk and macula to R/O abnormalities
11) Check BP
12) Check blood glucose

C) Assessment
1) 3-step test to isolate a paretic muscle in a vertical deviation. Neutralize by cover test or ask the patient to estimate the distance between the diplopic images in different fields of gaze
    a) Straight gaze: right hyperdeviation
        1) Right gaze: more hyperdeviation
            a) Right head tilt: more hyper = left inferior oblique
            b) Left head tilt: more hyper = right inferior rectus

        2) Left gaze: more hyperdeviation
           a) Right head tilt: more hyper = right superior oblique
           b) Left head tilt: more hyper = left superior rectus
      b) Straight gaze: left hyperdeviation
        1) Right gaze: more hyperdeviation
           a) Right head tilt: more hyper = right superior rectus
           b) Left head tilt: more hyper = left superior oblique
        2) Left gaze: more hyperdeviation
           a) Right head tilt: more hyper = left inferior rectus
           b) Left head tilt: more hyper = right inferior oblique
    2) Myasthenia gravis cold compress test: improvement in ptosis after the application of a cold compress is diagnostic for myasthenia gravis
      a) Patient relaxes and focuses on target in primary gaze
      b) Measure apertures
      c) Close eyes for 2 min to rest muscles
      d) Open and remeasure the aperture
      e) Wait for the lid to droop to normal position
      f) Apply an ice pack (ice in a latex glove) to the closed eye for 2 min
      g) Remeasure the aperture
      h) A 2 mm increase from the previous **after rest** measurement is positive for myasthenia gravis
      i) Tensilon is contraindicated in heart disease patients
      j) The cold test may not detect myasthenia gravis if there is complete ptosis
    3) If diabetic: 6x risk of 6th nerve palsy
    4) If diabetic and high BP: 8x risk of 6th nerve palsy

D) Plan

    1) Binocular diplopia of sudden onset
      a) Intermittent diplopia may be caused by
        1) Decompensating phoria: orthoptics or prism
        2) Myasthenia gravis: first available consult with neurologist
        3) Early nerve palsy: see below
        4) GCA: see neurovascular vision loss (Chapter 15). Work up if >age 60
      b) Constant diplopia causes
        1) Orbital
           a) Graves: order CT or MRI and refer to internist
           b) Pseudotumor: order CT or MRI and refer to internist or neurologist
           c) Tumor: order CT or MRI and refer to neurologist
        2) Nerve palsy: isolated, pupil sparing 3rd, 4th, and 6th nerve palsies of sudden onset without history of trauma and <than 4 weeks old are usually microvascular in adults. A new 6th nerve palsy in a child without trauma is likely to be a tumor; refer for neurologic workup
           a) 3rd (oculomotor) nerve palsy with or without pain

      1) Dilated pupil: STAT referral to neurologist or emergency department for MRI or cerebral angiogram to R/O an aneurysm

      2) Normal pupils

        a) History of diabetes or cardiovascular disease: consult a neurologist to confirm microvascular cause

        b) Negative history of diabetes or cardiovascular disease: STAT blood glucose and/or glycosylated hemoglobin test to R/O occult diabetes. If no diabetes, STAT referral to neurologist or emergency department for MRI

  b) 4th (trochlear) nerve palsy on 3-step test without trauma, pain, temporal arteritis Sx or proptosis

      1) Diabetic: check BP, inform internist, counsel, patch as needed, RTC in 1 month

        a) May worsen for 2 weeks

        b) 1 – 3 months to recover

        c) MRI if any other neurologic Sx or does not resolve in 3 months

        d) 95% recover

      2) Non-diabetic: check BP

        a) If elevated, have treated and RTC in 1 month

        b) If normal BP, do MRI or consult

  c) 6th (abducens) nerve palsy: see 4th nerve notes; also

      1) Test hearing in each ear. Simultaneously hold hands by each ear of patient. Rub thumb and forefinger together on each side. Should be equal and normal hearing. If a hearing loss is found a tumor needs to be ruled out by MRI

      2) Test 5th nerve corneal sensation with a cotton wisp on each cornea and compare before using drops

  d) Neuromuscular palsy

      1) Myasthenia gravis: refer to neurologist

  e) Brain-caused palsy

      1) Skew deviations: vertical, originate in the brain. Refer to neurologist

      2) Intranuclear ophthalmoplegia: refer to neurologist

Notes

17

PUPILS

A) Subjective
   1) Vary, but include central or peripheral vision loss, with or without pain, sudden diplopia, sudden ptosis, pupil abnormalities

B) Objective
   1) VA and pinhole or best corrected VA
   2) Pupils: use a bright light and look carefully for
      a) Anisocoria
      b) Direct pupil response
      c) Consensual response
      d) Afferent pupillary defect or reverse afferent pupillary defect
      e) Near response
   3) Eye movements
   4) Cover test: with 3-step test for vertical diplopia (see assessment in Chapter 16)
   5) External: R/O exophthalmos, measure ptosis if present
   6) Use a Hertel ophthalmometer on all potential orbital problems
   7) Red cap test or monocular color vision testing for all cases of optic nerve problems or monocular vision loss without an ocular cause
   8) Confrontation visual fields on all patients, threshold (30°) or Goldmann fields when indicated
   9) Slit lamp
   10) DFE
      a) BIO with scleral depression if necessary to R/O retinal detachments
      b) Fundus lens evaluation of disk and macula to R/O abnormalities
   11) Take BP
   12) Check blood glucose to R/O diabetes

C) Assessment
   1) Afferent pupillary defect assessment of causes
      a) Retina defect (should be visible ophthalmoscopically)
      b) Optic nerve defect (diagnosis of exclusion)
   2) Anisocoria pupil assessment (without visible ocular cause such as iritis or trauma)

a) In bright light the dilated pupil is the abnormal one except in Horner's syndrome
b) In dim light the constricted pupil is the abnormal one
    1) Miosis, ipsilateral ptosis, and lack of sweating
        a) Horner's syndrome: lesion in sympathetic innervation to the iris dilator muscle in 1 eye. Administer these tests 24 hrs apart
            1) 4% cocaine will dilate a normal eye but not a Horner's eye. If positive, isolate with paredrine testing at least 24 hrs later
            2) Pre-ganglionic lesion: paredrine 1% dilates and there is an ipsilateral loss of sweating to the face
            3) Post-ganglionic lesion: paredrine 1% does not dilate and the loss of sweating only affects the forehead
    2) Miosis, bilateral with irregular pupils and intact near reflex and accommodation (light-near dissociation)
        a) Argyll Robertson syndrome: midbrain lesion due to MS, syphilis, trauma, neoplasm or encephalitis
            1) Anisocoria is greater in dark
            2) Re-dilation after moving light away is faster than in a tonic pupil
    3) Dilated, sluggish pupil without APD, reduced near reflex and accommodation. The near reflex is better than the light reflex
        a) Adie's tonic pupil: post ganglionic parasympathetic lesion
            1) Diluted pilocarpine 0.125% will cause constriction in a tonic pupil. Mix 1 drop of 1% pilocarpine with 7 drops of saline, then instill both eyes (OU). In a positive test, the Adie's pupil will become the smaller pupil
            2) An old Adie's pupil will not constrict to light, but will still react to 0.125% pilocarpine
    4) Dilated unilateral or bilateral and fixed pupil in an otherwise healthy patient
        a) Pharmacologic pupil block: usually a history of handling a drug
            1) Will not constrict with 0.125% pilocarpine (an Adie's tonic pupil will)
            2) Will not constrict with 1% pilocarpine (a 3rd nerve palsy will)
    5) Dilated bilateral pupils unresponsive to light but with a near reflex, accommodative weakness, upgaze palsy with nystagmus on attempted upgaze
        a) Parinaud's syndrome: dorsal midbrain tumor
    6) Physiologic anisocoria
        a) Anisocoria is the same in light or dark
        b) Normal pupillary reactions
        c) Usually no more than 1 mm difference

      7) 3rd nerve palsy, non-pupil sparing
         a) Associated 3rd nerve muscle palsy

D) Plan
    1) Pupil abnormalities
       a) Horner's: acute onset of symptoms necessitate a STAT referral
         1) Pre-ganglionic: neurology consult for head and neck MRI to R/O a stroke or tumor
         2) Post-ganglionic: internist consult and MRI of brain, orbits, and chest to R/O a lung tumor or other chest tumor, unless a recent surgery or injury to neck or chest explains Horner's
       b) Argyll Robertson pupil
         1) Order an FTA-ABS or RPR or VDRL for syphilis. Refer to internist
       c) Adie's tonic pupil
         1) Confirm the diagnosis, then follow routinely
         2) Pilocarpine 0.125% may be helpful for cosmesis and vision
       d) Pharmacologic pupil block: counsel and monitor
       e) Parinaud's syndrome: neurologic referral
       f) Physiologic anisocoria: monitor routinely
       g) Non-pupil sparing 3rd nerve palsy: STAT referral to emergency department or neurologist

Notes

18

OCULAR COMPLICATIONS OF SINUSITIS

A) Subjective
    1) Classically, the patient presents with a severe loss of vision and an obviously proptotic eye
    2) The patient may also have sinus symptoms
    3) It is possible that the patient may be completely asymptomatic

B) Objective
    1) VAs and pinhole VAs usually (but not always) will show severely decreased vision
    2) An afferent pupillary defect will be present if the optic nerve is sufficiently compromised
    3) Monocular color vision results may show a loss of color vision in the affected eye
    4) Visual field testing may show constricted fields in the affected eye
    5) Exophthalmometry may reveal some degree of proptosis
    6) Extraocular muscle testing usually shows a restriction of gaze
    7) Dilated fundus examination may show papilledema or pallor of optic nerve
    8) Transillumination of maxillary sinuses
        a) Darken room completely
        b) Press the transilluminator behind the inferior orbital rim while the patient looks up and tips head back with mouth open so you can see the palate
        c) Compare the red glow on each side of the palate. Reduced transillumination indicates sinusitis
    9) Transillumination of frontal and maxillary sinuses
        a) Darken room completely
        b) Press transilluminator behind the brow of each eye with lids closed while the patient looks down
        c) Compare the red glow from the frontal sinus area on each side. Reduced transillumination indicates sinusitis
    10) Radiological exploration
        a) Axial and sagittal MRI images are best if a tumor or other soft tissue disorder is suspected
        b) A coronal CT scan with axial reconstruction is recommended when sinusitis is suspected. The CT will more accurately diagnose subperiosteal abscesses

       c) Plain x-rays are of no use
  11) Surgical exploration
       a) Endoscopic sinusectomy with frozen sections

C) Assessment
  1) Differential diagnosis
       a) Optic nerve tumor
       b) Orbital tumor
       c) Subperiosteal abscess trapped between the nasal orbital wall and the loosely adjacent periostium
       d) Acute sinus infections: classification
          1) Inflammatory edema: edema of the eyelids with or without edema of the orbital contents. The swelling may result from impedance of the drainage of the blood flow from superior ophthalmic veins into the ethmoid vessels. This is caused by obstruction of the vessels by pressure
          2) Orbital cellulitis: diffuse edema of the orbital contents and actual infiltration of the adipose tissue by inflammatory cells and bacteria. There is no discrete abscess formation. There may be some impairment of visual acuities if the process continues
          3) Subperiosteal abscess: a collection of pus between the periorbita and the bony wall of the orbit. There is a well-defined area of swelling that displaces the orbital contents and globe in a lateral or downward direction
          4) Orbital abscess: a discrete collection of pus that forms within the orbital tissues and may result from a progressive and localized orbital cellulitis. Exophthalmos is more marked, as is chemosis. There is complete ophthalmoplegia and severe impairment of vision usually occurs
          5) Cavernous sinus thrombosis: the phlebitis extends further posteriorally into the cavernous sinus. This results in the progression of symptoms followed by appearance of symptoms in the other eye. Frank meningitis is frequently noted
          6) Posterior orbital cellulitis: this occurs when a relatively small amount of inflammatory material or swelling is trapped and applies pressure adjacent to the optic nerve in the confined bony space of the posterior orbit. There may be no symptoms!
       e) Idiopathic inflammatory pseudotumor of the orbit: a noninfectious, inflammatory process which can cause symptoms similar to orbital cellulitis
  2) Facts
       a) Posterior ethmoid and sphenoid air cells are intimately related to the optic nerve canal
       b) Optic nerve is vulnerable to adjacent sinusitis

D) Plan

1) If any orbital condition is suspected which is causing demonstrable vision loss, radiologic exploration is necessary
2) If sinusitis is diagnosed in addition to the orbital condition, STAT referral to an ear, nose and throat specialist is necessary
3) If an orbital tumor is diagnosed, an urgent referral to an ophthalmologist specializing in oncology is recommended

Notes

19

CRANIAL NERVE AND CEREBELLAR TESTING

A) Olfactory (smell) CN I (sensory)
1) Occlude one nostril and present a recognizable odor (such as chocolate, vanilla, coffee) to the other nostril
2) Noxious odors such as alcohol or ammonia may cause a painful reaction, which may be mistaken for an intact olfactory nerve

B) Optic nerve (sight) CN II (sensory)
1) Central Snellen acuity
2) Peripheral vision (confrontation or automated or Goldmann)
3) Monocular color vision (red cap, Ishihara, Farnsworth D-15)
4) Dilated examination of the optic nerve appearance
5) Swinging flashlight test for afferent pupillary defect

C) Oculomotor (superior rectus, inferior rectus, medial rectus, inferior oblique, pupil constriction, accommodation, levator muscle of the upper lid) CN III (motor)
1) Eye movement testing
2) External examination for ptosis
3) Pupil testing for efferent loss of pupil constriction

D) Trochlear (superior oblique) CN IV (motor)
1) Eye movement testing

E) Trigeminal (afferent for cornea and face and efferent for jaw muscles) CN V (sensory and motor)
1) Ophthalmic afferent division
   a) Corneal reflex with a cotton wisp, compare reactions between eyes
   b) Close eyes, touch above one eyebrow with sharp or dull end of pin, have patient report which end was used. Compare sensation on each side
2) Maxillary afferent division
   a) Close eyes, use sharp and dull ends of pin to touch skin in the maxillary area on each side; compare
3) Mandibular afferent division
   a) Close eyes, use sharp and dull ends of pin to touch skin in the mandibular area on each side; compare

    4) Mandibular efferent division
        a) Have patient clench jaw, palpate jaw muscle for symmetry
        b) Move jaw from side to side against your resistance

F) Abducens (lateral rectus) CN VI (motor)
    1) Eye movement testing

G) Facial (facial muscles) CN VII (motor and sensory)
    1) Ask patient to lift eyebrows and wrinkle forehead. Look for
       symmetry
    2) Ask patient to close eyes as tightly as possible and resist your
       efforts to forcibly open them. Look for symmetry of strength
    3) Ask patient to smile, look for symmetry

H) Acoustic (auditory) CN VIII (sensory)
    1) Have patient close eyes; place your hand near each ear. Rub your
       thumb and finger together to make a small noise by one ear.
       Have patient report in which ear noise is heard. Repeat for the
       other ear. Look for symmetry
    2) Have patient close eyes and move a vibrating tuning fork near one
       ear until it is heard and then repeat for the other ear; compare
       hearing acuity
    3) Place the faintly vibrating tuning fork base on the mastoid bone
       and have the patient report when it is no longer heard. Then
       quickly place the fork near the same ear and ask if it can be heard
         a) Yes is normal
         b) No means a blockage of the ear canal (conduction loss)
    4) Place the faintly vibrating tuning fork base on the center of the
       forehead. Ask if the sound is heard more loudly on one side or the
       other
         a) Heard equally is normal
         b) Heard more loudly on the side with decreased hearing
           indicates bone conduction deficit
         c) Heard more loudly on the opposite side from the one with
           decreased hearing indicates a neural deficit

**I) Glossopharyngeal (taste, salivation, afferent) CN IX (sensory and
   motor)**
    1) Open patient's mouth, look for symmetry of arches of palate
    2) Touch palate with tongue depressor; look for gagging
    3) Ask about trouble with speech and swallowing

**J) Vagus (efferent muscles of speech and swallowing, also
   autonomic nerves to chest and abdomen) CN X (sensory and
   motor)**
    1) Open patient's mouth, look for symmetry of arches of palate
    2) Touch palate with tongue depressor; look for symmetric elevation
       of palate

    3) Ask about trouble with speech and swallowing

K) Accessory (moves the head and elevates shoulders) CN XI (motor)
    1) Hold down shoulders and have the patient elevate them against your resistance. Look for strength and symmetry
    2) Hold patient's head and have him/her turn it against your resistance. Look for strength and symmetry

L) Hypoglossal (moves the tongue) CN XII (motor)
    1) Have the patient stick out tongue. If there is a weakness, tongue will deviate toward the weak side

M) Cerebellar function
    1) Finger to nose: patient extends one arm to the side with eyes closed, then touches the nose with eyes closed. Repeat with the other arm. Look for tremor or inaccuracy
    2) Knee pat: the seated patient pats his/her knees alternately with the palms and backs of the hands slowly, then gradually increases to maximum speed. Look for speed, rhythm, or position

Notes____

20

MALINGERING AND HYSTERIA

A) Subjective
- 1) Adults
  - a) Claimed loss of central or peripheral vision
  - b) May be involved in insurance claims or recent accidents or trauma
- 2) Children
  - a) Unlikely to complain of a loss of peripheral vision
  - b) If asked, grade school age children will frequently state that a friend has recently been given glasses

B) Objective: vision is reduced with no visible reason such as pathology or amblyogenic factors
- 1) Claimed monocular loss of VA (children usually claim binocular loss)
  - a) Claimed hand motion or worse vision
    - 1) Afferent pupillary defect should be present if the loss is physiologic
    - 2) Optokinetic drum or strip: optokinetic nystagmus absent in physiologic loss
    - 3) Patch the good eye and make some pretense to have the patient move from one room to another, etc. True vision loss at this level will cause difficulty with navigation. Be prepared to prevent injury if the loss is true
  - b) Claimed vision of 20/40 – 20/400
    - 1) Isolate a single letter at distance 1 line bigger than best-claimed VA in the **good** eye and ask the patient to read it. Then insert a 4 pd base down prism in front of the good eye and ask what is seen
      - a) If the patient still sees only 1 letter that moved, there is a functional vision loss
      - b) If the patient sees 2 letters, the vision in the poorer eye is at least as good as the size of the letter shown
    - 2) Persistently encourage the patient to try harder to read the successive lines through the phoropter with the best refraction or retinoscopy results dialed in. Works best for children

      3) Dial fogging lens in and out rapidly for each eye to try to trick into losing track of which eye is "blind"

      4) Use dissociating prism rapidly to trick into reading before patient can determine which eye is seeing

      5) Red, green or Polaroid filters: when the chart is presented with letters one size larger than the claimed best vision, physiologic loss will only allow the patient to read half of the chart. Do not allow the patient time to figure out which eye can see each part of the chart

      6) Cover the "good" eye and lead half way to the letter chart. Or preferably switch to a hand held distance chart at 10 ft to make it difficult for a malingerer to determine what line to read. If the loss is physiologic, the patient should be able to read letters half the size as at 20 ft. Malingering/hysterical patients read the same row as before

      7) Test near vision; if normal and no myopia is present, diagnose malingering

  2) Claimed binocular loss of VA

    a) Claimed hand motion or worse VA

      1) Optokinetic drum test: nystagmus indicates better than hand motion vision

      2) Observe the patient surreptitiously; this level of vision should seriously hamper mobility

    b) Claimed vision of 20/40 – 20/400

      1) Persistently encourage patient to read the next line. Works best for kids and hysterics

      2) Move up to half of the usual distance to the acuity chart, or preferably use a hand held distance chart at 10 ft instead of 20 ft

      3) Test near vision; if normal and no myopia is present, diagnose malingering

  3) Claimed loss of peripheral vision

    a) Typically claim "tunnel vision" as opposed to more common hemianopsia and scotoma

    b) Test peripheral vision with counting fingers, or preferably with a tangent screen, at standard distance. Repeat test at double the distance. Physiologic loss will give a seeing area of approximately twice the diameter at twice the distance. Malingerers will report a seeing area about the same diameter at twice the distance

    c) On automated testing the diameter of seen field is the same with different visibility targets, yielding a normal central area surrounded by completely unseeing area

C) Assessment

  1) R/O all ophthalmic and neurologic causes that you can with in-office testing such as

    a) Strabismic amblyopia: cover testing

    b) Refractive amblyopia: cycloplegic refraction or retinoscopy
    c) Retrobulbar optic neuritis: afferent pupillary defect if large vision loss; also do monocular color vision testing or red cap testing
    d) Space occupying lesions of head: visual field testing should yield neurologic pattern
    e) Keratoconus: do keratometry or corneal topography
    f) Do a careful slit lamp and ophthalmoscopy, including a contact lens evaluation of the macula if necessary to R/O pathology

2) Factors indicating malingering
    a) Inquire about the circumstances of the loss. Adults typically are involved in an insurance claim or accident
    b) Children usually have a friend who was recently given desirable glasses, or they may have unresolved problems at school or at home, looking for attention
    c) A plano lens may improve acuity
    d) Asthenopia may be claimed
    e) Patient may be uncooperative
    f) Exaggerated orientation difficulties may be claimed

3) Factors indicating hysteria
    a) More likely to be females <age 30
    b) Larger letters are read as tentatively as small letters
    c) Acuity may be improved by suggestion
    d) The patient may be overly cooperative
    e) No orientation difficulty

D) Plan for hysterics or malingerers

1) Assure children you found a little problem but that you will cure it with some strong medicine. Instill dilating drops and retest vision after cycloplegic retinoscopy and refraction. This gives them an honorable way out of their deception
2) Assure patients their eyes are fine and you expect them to be seeing much better by the time of their next visit
3) RTC in 2 weeks and retest
4) If doubt about diagnosis, consider MRI, CT, electroretinography (ERG), FANG
5) For hysterics, a mental health referral may be indicated

Notes____

____

____

____

____

____

21

MENTAL STATUS EXAMINATION

A) Subjective
1) Alertness: consciousness or wakefulness
2) Orientation to
   a) Person: who you are
   b) Place: where you are
   c) Time: day or date
3) Mood or affect: patient's tone or feeling expressed vocally or by demeanor and appearance
4) Attention: is the patient able to attend to a conversation and does the conversation display normal sequence, logic, coherence and relevance?
5) Intellect: is the patient's knowledge and vocabulary consistent with their education or occupation?
6) Memory
   a) Short term
   b) Long term

B) Objective: short portable mental status questionnaire
1) What is the date today?
2) What day of the week is it?
3) Where are we right now?
4) What is your telephone number?
5) How old are you?
6) When were you born?
7) Who is the President of the United States?
8) Who was the President just before that?
9) What is your mother's maiden name?
10) Subtract 3 from 20 and keep subtracting 3 from each new number until you get all the way down

C) Assessment
1) For patients with a high school education
   a) 0 – 2 errors = intact mental function
   b) 3 – 4 errors = mild mental impairment
   c) 5 – 7 errors = moderate mental impairment
   d) 8 – 10 errors = severe mental impairment
2) For grade school education, allow one more error

3) For post high school education, allow one less error

D) Plan
1) Note findings in your record
2) For billing higher level medical exams, your record should state if the patient is alert and oriented to person, place, and time. Also, whether the patient's mood and affect is normal; this can be a subjective judgment on your part
3) If you diagnose mental impairment in a patient not already under treatment, refer for further evaluation and treatment

Notes____

22

SELECTIVE LASER TRABECULOPLASTY OR ARGON LASER TRABECULOPLASTY POST-OP CARE

All post-op co-management should be coordinated with the surgeon, using his/her protocols and recommendations. This section is a guide to use in the absence of this coordination.

A) Subjective at 1 or 2 day post-op

1) There should be no change in vision or comfort since the laser. Patient may have had some irritation the day of the procedure from the gonioscopy laser lens
2) Patient should still be on all pre-op glaucoma meds OU plus Pred Forte (or equivalent steroid) 3 – 4x in the treated eye

B) Objective

1) VA: should be unchanged
2) Slit lamp: there may be mild cell or flare or pigment in the AC
3) IOP: may be up or down some from pre-op measurements
4) Gonioscopy: the treated part of the trabecular meshwork should have about 50 mildly blanched spots per 180° with ALT. There should be no anterior synechiae or hemorrhages

C) Assessment/Plan

1) Inflammation
   a) Quiet AC: instruct to taper off the steroid by 4 days post-op. RTC in 1 month. You should have IOP lowering by then to allow you to either hit a lower target IOP or to discontinue 1 medication
   b) Cell or flare in the AC: continue the steroid drop or even increase if necessary and RTC in 2 – 3 days
2) IOP: no IOP drop is expected for about 1 month and may even spike in the immediate post-op period
   a) IOP approximately the same or less than pre-op: continue same glaucoma meds at this time
   b) IOP up significantly
      1) If no cell or flare: discontinue steroid and RTC in 2 days
      2) If significant cell or flare: increase steroid because inflammation of the trabecular meshwork may be causing

an IOP spike. If the optic nerve is threatened, increase glaucoma meds at this time. RTC in 2 – 3 days

Notes

23

CATARACT SURGERY WITH POSTERIOR CHAMBER IOL POST-OP CARE

All post-op co-management should be coordinated with the surgeon, using his/her protocols and recommendations. This section is a guide to use in the absence of this coordination. This guide assumes one of the modern phakoemulsification techniques with a small incision. There may be 1 or no sutures.

A) Subjective at 1 or 2 day post-op
    1) Vision is usually described as "brighter" at this point, even though it may not be clear yet
    2) A foreign body or scratchy sensation is expected. There may be some deep tenderness if a retrobulbar injection was used. There should not have been enough pain to interfere with sleep
    3) The patient should be on a topical antibiotic, steroid, and possibly a non-steroidal anti-inflammatory qid in the operated eye. Patient may be patched or have been wearing a protective shield while sleeping

B) Objective
    1) Pinhole VA: may or may not be improved yet
    2) If you are concerned about post-op corneal cylinder and do not want to refract yet, do keratometry instead
    3) External and slit lamp
        a) Expect a mild ptosis, injection, subconjunctival hemorrhage and lid bruising
        b) The cornea will have at least mild striae up to frank folds depending on the surgeon's technique. The wound in the cornea or limbus should be closed with no Seidel's sign. Sutures, if present, should be buried with no exposed barbs
        c) There is usually cell or flare or pigment in the AC
        d) Pupil should be round
        e) IOL should be approximately centered. Posterior capsule should be intact and clear
        f) There should be no vitreous prolapse
    4) IOP: should be similar to pre-op measurements

5) DFE: look carefully for any peripheral holes or tears as well as for macular edema. The posterior chamber should be clear and quiet with no sign of endophthalmitis. Dilation may be postponed to the 1 week visit

C) Assessment/Plan
1) Inflammation
   a) Up to 1+ cell and flare in the AC: instruct to continue post-op medications as instructed by the surgeon; RTC in 1 week
   b) Greater than 1+ cell or flare or hypopyon in the AC, or vitreous inflammation, call the surgeon and consult. Expected inflammation varies by surgeon and technique
2) Wound: should be closed; if Seidel's sign is present, call the surgeon
3) Macular edema is rarely expected with modern techniques but should respond to Pred Forte and Voltaren drops qid
4) Corneal striae are expected and should resolve over time
5) Send a timely report to the co-managing surgeon

D) Continuing follow up
1) In normal healing RTC at 1 week, 3 weeks and 6 weeks. With clear corneal incision and a good technique, RTC at 1 week and 1 month
2) Do the DFE at 1 week if not done at 1 day. In routine cases, 1 DFE is sufficient during the post-op period
3) Prescribe glasses when refraction is stabilized and corneal edema is resolved
4) Repeat all of the other above-listed history and testing at each visit
   a) Discomfort should be mostly gone by 1 week
   b) All objective findings should gradually resolve
   c) Pinhole or corrected vision should gradually improve to expected levels based on edema, inflammation and macular function. If there is a problem, call the surgeon
   d) Modify the post-op medication regimen as needed according to healing response
   e) Always send reports to the surgeon
5) Have patient follow the post-op instructions regarding heavy lifting and wearing the eye shield. This varies according to the surgical technique used
6) When out of the post-op period, RTC at 6 – 12 months to monitor for capsular opacification or other eye changes

Notes____

____

____

____

24

LASIK Post-Op Care

All post-op co-management should be coordinated with the surgeon using his/her protocols and recommendations. This section is a guide to use in the absence of this coordination.

A) Subjective at 1 or 2 day post-op
1) Vision will be better than pre-op, but is likely to still be blurry, especially at near
2) Some foreign body or dry eye sensation may remain
3) Patient should be taking topical antibiotic and steroid drops, approximately qid, tears prn and possibly a non-steroidal anti-inflammatory drop qid

B) Objective
1) Distance VA may range from 20/20 – 20/100 due to temporary hyperopia. Larger corrections result in more overcorrection at this point. Accommodative reserve predicts VA
2) Pinhole VA should be near 20/20 – 20/30
3) Slit lamp
   a) Note and draw any subconjunctival hemorrhages (which are common)
   b) Look carefully at the flap. It should be centered and have no gross wrinkles. Micro striae may be present
   c) Note and draw any epithelial defects or staining
   d) Note and draw any opacities in the flap interface
   e) Note and draw any sign of epithelial ingrowth
   f) Be sure the AC is quiet

C) Assessment
1) If the flap is well centered and flat and there is no sign of infection, everything is OK at this stage

D) Plan
1) If there is a flap problem, call the surgeon immediately
2) If there is any sign of infiltrate or infection, use Vigamox q1h and notify the surgeon
3) Metallic glistenings noted at the flap interface can be ignored

    4) If there is evidence of inflammation in the interface (haze, sands of the Sahara), start Pred Forte q1h
    5) Counsel that VA will improve, consider using inexpensive reading glasses
    6) Counsel that dry eye Sx will resolve, use lubrication qid or more until then. Some experts think that frequent lubrication helps the healing process regardless of dry eye symptoms
    7) Remind the patient to continue to sleep with an eye shield on for the next week
    8) Send report to the surgeon

E) Continuing follow up: 1 week
    1) Vision should be improving but fluctuation is expected
    2) Refract, expect mild hyperopia; expect 20/20 best corrected
    3) Cornea should look normal except for mild flap interface debris and micro striae
    4) IOP: normal or lower
    5) Antibiotics can be discontinued
    6) Steroids should be continued if flap inflammation is present
    7) Send report to the surgeon

F) Continuing follow up: 1 month
    1) Symptoms should be nearly normal with little fluctuation in vision, glare or halos
    2) Refract, expect 20/20 best corrected vision
    3) Cornea should be normal except for mild flap interface debris and micro striae
    4) Be sure there is no epithelial ingrowth in the wound. Send back to the surgeon if it is growing or threatens the flap or vision
    5) Send report to the surgeon

G) Continuing follow up: 3 months
    1) Sx should be normal at this time in lower corrections. High corrections may still have some glare and halos
    2) Refract, consider myopic enhancement if residual error and perceived blur are significant (*i.e.*, usually >- 0.75)
    3) Slit lamp results should be normal except for mild flap interface debris and micro striae
    4) Prescribe over-correction if needed
    5) Send report to the surgeon

H) Continuing follow up: 6 months
    1) All Sx and objective findings should have stabilized by this time
    2) Hyperopic enhancements or secondary myopic corrections may be done now
    3) Send report to the surgeon

I) Continuing follow up: 1 yr and yearly thereafter
    1) Perform a normal eye exam including dilated fundus examination

2) Remind the patient of the need for yearly eye exams even if his/her vision is 20/20: especially if the patient was a high myope previously
3) Remember that corneal thinning reduces IOP by about 1 mmHg per 20 microns after LASIK

Notes

25

LASER PERIPHERAL IRIDOTOMY

All post-op co-management should be coordinated with the surgeon, using his/her protocols and recommendations. This section is a guide to use in the absence of this coordination.

A) Subjective at 1 or 2 day post-op
1) There should be no change in comfort since the laser. Vision should be the same. They may have had some irritation the day of the procedure from the laser lens
2) Patient should still be on all pre-op eye meds (if any) OU plus Pred Forte (or equivalent steroid) 3 – 4x in the treated eye

B) Objective
1) VA: should be unchanged and up to the level expected by the health of the eye
2) Slit lamp: there may be mild cell, flare, or pigment in the AC. There should be a visible hole in the superior iris that can be retro illuminated. Also, look with direct illumination; be sure there is no membrane covering the hole. The angle should be noticeably deeper
3) IOP: should be similar or possibly lower than pre-op measurements
4) DFE: look carefully for any peripheral holes or tears

C) Assessment/Plan
1) Inflammation
    a) Quiet AC: instruct to taper off steroid by 4 days post-op, RTC in 6 – 12 months
    b) Cell or flare in the AC: continue steroid drop or even increase if necessary and RTC in 2 – 3 days
2) IOP
    a) IOP approximately the same or less than pre-op, RTC in 6 – 12 months
    b) IOP significantly greater
        1) If no cell or flare: discontinue steroid and RTC in 2 days
        2) If significant cell or flare: increase steroid because inflammation may be causing an IOP spike. If the optic

nerve is threatened, start or increase glaucoma meds at this time. RTC in 2 – 3 days

c) Watch for future IOP rises. Many of these patients develop open angle glaucoma

Notes

26

YAG Capsulotomy Post-Op Care

All post-op co-management should be coordinated with the surgeon using his/her protocols and recommendations. This section is a guide to use in the absence of this coordination.

A) Subjective at 1 or 2 day post-op
1) There should be no change in comfort since the laser. Vision should be noticeably better. There may have been some irritation the day of the procedure from the laser lens
2) Patient should still be on all pre-op eye meds (if any) OU plus Pred Forte (or equivalent steroid) 3 – 4x in the treated eye

B) Objective
1) VA: should be improved and up to the level expected by the eye health
2) Slit lamp: there may be mild cell, flare, or pigment in the AC. There should be a capsular hole at least the size of the natural pupil. Some pits may be visible in the IOL. IOL should not have moved or decentered
3) IOP: should be similar to pre-op measurements
4) DFE: look carefully for any peripheral holes or tears as well as for macular edema

C) Assessment/Plan
1) Inflammation
   a) Quiet AC: instruct to taper off steroid by 4 days post-op. RTC in 6 – 12 months
   b) Cell or flare in AC: continue the steroid drop or even increase if necessary and RTC in 2 – 3 days
2) IOP
   a) IOP approximately the same or less than pre-op, RTC in 6 – 12 months
   b) IOP up significantly
      1) If no cell or flare: discontinue steroid and RTC in 2 days
      2) If significant cell or flare: increase steroid because inflammation may be causing an IOP spike. If optic nerve is threatened, start or increase glaucoma meds at this time. RTC in 2 – 3 days

Notes

27

THE PEDIATRIC EYE EXAMINATION
Chapters 27 – 31 by Valerie M. Kattouf, OD, FAAO

A) Summary of the infant eye examination
1) Gross visual acuity measure (preferential looking as needed)
2) Extra ocular muscles (EOM)/motilities (fixate and follow)
3) Vergence = near point of convergence (NPC)
4) Alignment
- a) Hirschberg/Kappa
- b) Bruckner test
5) Pupils
6) Refraction = cycloplegic retinoscopy
7) Anterior segment evaluation
8) Dilated exam/posterior pole evaluation

B) Summary of the preschool eye examination
1) Visual acuity symbols
2) Motilities
3) Cover test (accommodative target)
4) Vergence
- a) NPC
- b) Prism bar vergences as needed
- c) Accommodative testing as needed
  - 1) Pull away amplitudes
  - 2) Monocular estimation method retinoscopy (MEM)
5) Random dot stereopsis
6) Color Vision Made Easy
7) Refraction
- a) Dry/Mohindra retinoscopy
- b) Cycloplegic retinoscopy
8) Pupils
9) Anterior segment evaluation
- a) 20 D Lens
- b) Hand held slit lamp
10) Dilated exam/posterior segment evaluation

C) Case history
1) Ocular history
- a) Chief complaint

      b) Previous ocular diagnosis and treatments
         1) Glasses and/or contact lenses
            a) When started?
            b) How old is current pair?
         2) Patching and/or vision therapy
            a) Type?
            b) How long?
            c) Compliance?
         3) Surgery (type and date)
         4) Other problems (cataracts, retinopathy of prematurity
           (ROP), glaucoma, etc.)
  2) Birth history
     a) Full term?
        1) How many weeks premature?
        2) Premature = <than 37 weeks
     b) Birth weight?/normal ≥ 5 lbs 5 oz
     c) Delivery complications
        1) Need for oxygen after birth?
        2) If yes, how long? (determines risk of retinopathy of
          prematurity)
     d) Developmental history
        1) Normal/delayed
        2) Is the child undergoing occupational, physical,
          developmental or speech therapy?
  3) Medical history
     a) Current medication
     b) Allergies to medications
     c) Review of systems
  4) Family ocular history
     a) High refractive error
     b) Strabismus/amblyopia
     c) Other family eye diseases

D) VA assessment
  1) Non-quantitative visual acuity assessment (infants and non-verbal
    patients)
     a) Fixate and follow (F&F): target transilluminator or small toy
       (without auditory component)
       1) Binocularly (same as extraocular motility assessment)
       2) Monocularly: compare ability to track target OD vs. OS
     b) Optokinetic drum
       1) Working distance 5 – 10 cm, slow rotation
       2) Watch for brisk nystagmus in response to stripes on drum
         (may attempt horizontally and vertically)
       3) Goal: predicts visual resolution up to, but not including, the
         visual cortex
     c) 10 Δ base down test
       1) Place 10 Δ base down prism over one eye
       2) Hold transilluminator 50 cm from patient in dimly lit room

       3) Observe for spontaneous alternation of fixation in response to diplopia created by the prism
       4) Interpretation of (+) alternation = patient is not suppressing, ↓ likelihood of amblyopia
       5) Interpretation of (-) alternation = patient is suppressing, ↑ likelihood of amblyopia OR patient simply not responding to procedure
       6) Goal: assesses presence of a fixation preference to R/O monocular amblyopia
    d) Candy bead test (recommend use small cake-decorating sprinkles)
       1) Place 1 candy piece in palm of examiner's hand
       2) Patient occluded by parent/adhesive occlusion
       3) Observe visually directed reaching ability with right eye viewing
       4) Observe visually directed reaching ability with left eye viewing
       5) Monitor for a difference in behavior/performance/ability with either eye viewing
       6) Eye with more difficulty may represent ↑ likelihood of amblyopia/pathology
  2) Quantitative VA assessment (directions included with test/see Chapter 27 Appendix for suppliers)
    a) Preferential looking (children age 3 months – 12 months)
    b) Lea symbols (age 3 and up)
    c) HOTV (age 3 and up)
    d) Broken wheel (age 3 and up)

E) Ocular motility examination (system fully developed at 3 – 4 months)
  1) Position maintenance/fixation
  2) Smooth pursuits
  3) Saccades: evaluate each (1 – 3) with an age-appropriate target
    a) Transilluminator: infants (hold head)
    b) Toy (without auditory component): toddler (hold head)
    c) Pediatric target
       1) *e.g.*, detailed sticker: school age
       2) Determine if capable of eye-head dissociation

F) Refractive error assessment
  1) Retinoscopy: increased effectiveness when performed out of phoropter, use lens bars or trial lenses
    a) Mohindra retinoscopy technique (technique for children ~ 5 yrs old and under)
       1) Dark room/50 cm working distance
       2) Patient is monocular
       3) Patient fixates retinoscope light
       4) Neutralize primary meridians

     5) Transpose to spherocylindrical form

     6) Subtract 1.25 from sphere power

     7) Goal: to control accommodation without the use of diagnostic agents

  b) Cycloplegic retinoscopy

     1) Administration of cycloplegic agents (for proper cycloplegic refraction and dilation)

       a) Drops

         1) 1 gtt cyclopentolate

- 1.0% >1 yr old
- 0.5% <1 yr old

         2) 1 gtt tropicamide

- 1.0% >1 yr old
- 0.5% <1 yr old

         3) 2.5% Neo-Synephrine

       b) Spray for increased ease of installation in pediatric population (see Chapter 27 Appendix for ordering information)

         1) Combination #1: children >1 yr old

            a) 1.0% cyclopentolate

            b) 1.0% tropicamide

            c) 2.5% Neo-Synephrine

         2) Combination #2: children <1 yr old

            a) 0.5% cyclopentolate

            b) 0.5% tropicamide

            c) 2.5% Neo-Synephrine

     2) Indications for a cycloplegic exam

       a) Esotropia (ET)(any new patient)

       b) Moderate to high hyperopia

       c) New patients <5 yrs old

       d) Uncooperative/non-communicative patient

       e) Acuity not corrected to predicted level

       f) Suspected malingering

       g) Suspected hysterical amblyopia

2) Additional methods of assessment of refractive error in pediatric patients

  a) Keratometry (hand held available for young patients)

  b) Auto refractor (only reliable if child is under effect of cyclopentolate)

3) Prescribing guidelines for children

  a) The highest rate of emmetropization takes place in the first 12 – 17 months

  b) Hyperopia

     1) The average refractive error in infants is +2.00 D of hyperopia

     2) Children with greater than 1.50 D of hyperopia at 5 yrs old often remain hyperopic

  c) Myopia

        1) 25% of infants are myopic
            a) Approximately 50% of these remain myopic
            b) Approximately 50% of these become emmetropic
      d) Astigmatism
        1) Against-the-rule astigmatism more prevalent at birth and switches to with-the-rule with development
        2) At 3 ½ yrs old astigmatism is at adult levels

G) Assessment of vergence/accommodation/stereopsis/color vision
    1) All of the above visual systems are fully functional at 3 – 4 months of age
    2) Vergence testing
      a) Near point of convergence
        1) Norm = break (diplopia) at 6 cm
      b) Prism bar vergences (step): age 5 and older
        1) Norms for children 7 – 12 yrs old
          a) Base out (near)
            • Break = 23
            • Recovery = 16
          b) Base in (near)
            • Break = 12
            • Recovery = 7
    3) Accommodative testing
      a) Push up/pull away testing: age 5 and older
        1) Use equivalent of 20/30 target (recommend pull away as a more objective measure)
        2) Child is occluded with eyes closed
        3) Place target at spectacle plane, have child open eyes
        4) Pull target away until child verbally names target
        5) Measure test distance with a PD rule
        6) Divide distance in cm into 100 = dioptric value
        7) Minimum amplitude norms = 15 –¼ age
      b) MEM
        1) Use age-appropriate MEM cards mounted on retinoscope
        2) Child verbally calls out pictures/words
        3) Examiner performs retinoscopy on each principal meridian
        4) Document on optical cross
          • Using age appropriate target
          • Norms = +0.25 D to +0.50 D
    4) Stereopsis testing
      a) Needing stereo glasses
        1) Randot stereo fly = peripheral stereopsis
        2) Randot circles = lateral disparity
        3) Randot animals = lateral disparity
        4) Randot forms = random dot
      b) Without stereo glasses (beneficial for young children)
        1) Lang stereopsis: random dot

      c) Note: random dot stereopsis is the only type of stereopsis that confirms bifixation

   5) Color vision testing

      a) Ishihara: school age children

      b) Color Vision Made Easy (see Chapter 27 Appendix): toddlers

H) Detection of strabismus in the pediatric population

   1) Bruckner test

      a) Appropriate for infants and toddlers

      b) Goal: detects as little as 2 Δ of strabismus

      c) Procedure

         1) Use direct ophthalmoscope at 1M from patient

         2) Room is dark/patient looks at light

         3) Look through the scope as you shine the light at the bridge of the patient's nose

         4) With the patient optically corrected, look at the orange-red retinal reflexes

         5) Compare the color and brightness between the 2 eyes simultaneously

         6) Record

            a) (+) Bifixation if retinal reflexes are equal in appearance

            b) If a whiter and brighter reflex exists, note which eye; this is the STRABISMIC EYE

   2) Hirschberg/Kappa test

      a) Appropriate for infants and toddlers, patients with a monocular reduction in visual acuity or poor attentiveness/fixation

      b) Goal: determines laterality, direction and frequency of strabismus

      c) Procedure

         1) Step I: Hirschberg

            a) Patient is **binocular**

            b) Shine light at bridge of nose as patient fixates transilluminator

            c) Evaluate placement of the binocular corneal reflexes in relation to the center of the pupil OD and OS

            d) Follow with <Kappa

         2) Step II: Kappa

             a) Patient is monocular

             b) Shine light at bridge of nose as patient fixates transilluminator

            c) Evaluate placement of the monocular corneal reflexes in relation to the center of the pupil OD and OS

            d) Compare to Hirschberg results

         3) Interpretation of Hirschberg/Kappa

            a) Hirschberg reflexes (binocular) = Kappa reflexes (monocular), no strabismus exists

        b) Hirschberg reflexes (binocular) ≠ Kappa reflexes (monocular), strabismus exists, Kappa determines the fixating eye

        c) Light reflex placement

           1) Nasal light reflex = exotropia

           2) Temporal light reflex = esotropia

           3) Superior light reflex = hypotropia

           4) Inferior light reflex = hypertropia

3) Krimsky test

    a) Appropriate for infants and toddlers, patients with a monocular reduction in visual acuity or poor attentiveness/fixation

    b) Goal: determines magnitude of strabismus

    c) Procedure

        1) Perform Hirschberg, view corneal light reflexes

        2) Place prism in front of non-strabismic eye

        3) Add prism until the corneal reflex in the deviating eye looks symmetrical with that of the fixating eye

        4) The amount of prism necessary to achieve this = the magnitude of the strabismic deviation

4) Cover test

    a) Appropriate for any child able to hold fixation

    b) Mandatory for any child 3 yrs of age and older

    c) Goal: determines presence/absence of strabismus

    d) Procedure: must use accommodative targets in this age group. Age-appropriate targets

        1) Toddler = detailed sticker on a tongue depressor

        2) School age

           a) Detailed sticker on a tongue depressor

           b) Appropriate-size letter

        3) Perform unilateral cover test (UCT) to determine

           a) Phoria vs. strabismus

           b) Laterality of strabismus, if present

           c) Frequency of strabismus, if present

        4) Perform alternating cover test (ACT) to determine the magnitude of strabismus or phoria

I) Anterior segment examination of the pediatric patient

1) Anterior segment normative values

    a) Corneal horizontal diameter

        1) Neonate = 9 mm

        2) 1 yr old = 10 mm

        3) 3 – 4 yrs old = 11.5 mm: 12.0 mm (adult level)

    b) Pupils

        1) Size

           a) Resting = 2.5 mm – 4.0 mm

           b) Constricted = 1.2 mm – 2.0 mm

           c) Fully dilated = 7.5 mm – 8.0 mm

        2) Reaction

           a) Less in infancy than in childhood

        b) Often absent in premature children
2) Anterior segment examination technique
    a) Biomicroscope/slit lamp if child is age and size appropriate
        1) Hint: having a child sit on his/her knees gives examiner a better ability to fit and control the child in the slit lamp
    b) Hand-held slit lamp
    c) Burton lamp
    d) 20 D lens + transilluminator for magnification
    e) Sodium fluorescein (NaFl) staining when necessary
        1) Blue filter on slit lamps and Burton lamp
        2) Blue filter on direct ophthalmoscope + 20 D lens
3) IOP measurement: Tono-Pen
    a) Norms are 8 – 15 mmHg
    b) Increases by 1 mmHg/yr from birth – 5 yrs old

J) Posterior segment examination of the pediatric patient
1) Posterior segment normative values
    a) Vascularization of the infant retina
        1) Nasal retina = 32 weeks gestation
        2) Temporal retina = 40 – 42 weeks gestation
    b) Macula fully developed at 42 weeks
2) Posterior segment examination technique
    a) BIO
        1) Posterior pole only view likely on most healthy infants/toddlers
        2) Peripheral views can be obtained on school-age children who can fixate

Chapter 27 Appendix

- Vision Associates
  4209 US Hwy 90 West
  #312
  Lake City, FL 32055
  (386) 752-7839
  www.visionkits.com
  (Infant visual acuity tests, Color Vision Made Easy, stereopsis tests, etc.)

- Richmond Products
  1021 S. Rogers Circle Suite #6
  Boca Raton, FL 33487-2894
  www.RichmondProducts.com
  (Infant visual acuity tests, Color Vision Made Easy, stereopsis tests, pediatric trial frames, pediatric fixation targets, pediatric occluders, etc.)

- Bernell Corporation
  750 Lincolnway East
  PO Box 4637
  South Bend, IN 46634
  (800) 348-2225
  www.bernell.com
  (Visual acuity, stereopsis tests, vision therapy equipment, etc.)

- Star Ophthalmic Instruments
  7101 Adams St. Suite 2
  Willowbrook, IL 60521
  (630) 655-4500
  www.starop.com
  (Skiascopy bars, diagnostic lenses, prism boxes, etc.)

- O'Brian Pharmacy
  (800) 627-4360
  (Cycloplegic spray)

Notes

28

DIAGNOSIS AND MANAGEMENT OF NEAR POINT BINOCULAR VISION PROBLEMS

CONVERGENCE EXCESS (CE)

A) Subjective
- 1) Symptoms associated with near work
  - a) Headaches
  - b) Asthenopia
  - c) Diplopia
  - d) Intermittent blur/print moves on page
  - e) Fatigue
  - f) Avoidance of near tasks
  - g) May demonstrate poor reading skills relative to intelligence

B) Objective
- 1) Cover test
  - a) High eso deviation at near (near >distance)
    - 1) Normal lateral phoria value = $6 - 8\ \Delta$ exophoria
    - 2) May break down into intermittent esotropia with fatigue and/or prolonged dissociation
- 2) Fusional vergences
  - a) Near base in (BI)/negative fusional vergences low in convergence excess (CE) patients
  - b) Near base out (BO)/positive fusional vergences normal to high in CE patients
  - c) Vergence norms
    - 1) Step/prism bar vergences
      - a) Adults (break/recovery)
        - 1) Near BO = 19/14
        - 2) Near BI = 13/10
      - b) Children 7 – 12 yrs (break/recovery)
        - 1) Near BO = 23/16
        - 2) Near BI = 12/7
    - 2) Smooth/phoropter vergences
      - a) All ages (blur/break/recovery)
        - 1) Near BO = 17/21/11

        2) Near BI = 13/21/13
    d) Compensating vergences based on Sheard's criteria
        1) Break = 2x phoria [see patient example in **D) Plan,** 5)
           Treatment tips below]
  3) High accommodative convergence/accommodation (AC/A) ratio
    a) Normal value = 4/1
  4) Stereopsis usually adequate
    a) Wirt circles
    b) Random dot
    c) If absent, patient may exhibit strabismus/intermittent esotropia
      at near
  5) Accommodative facility testing (using +/- 2.00 D binocular flippers)
    a) Cannot clear minus lenses secondary to poor divergence

C) Assessment
  1) Summary of typical finding
    a) High eso deviation at near
    b) Low BI vergence ranges
    c) High AC/A ratio
    d) Adequate stereopsis
    e) Inability to clear minus lenses binocularly
  2) Differential diagnosis
    a) Uncorrected refractive error
        1) Perform cycloplegic retinoscopy to R/O hyperopia,
           pseudomyopia, etc.
    b) Other eso classifications
        1) Divergence insufficiency
           a) Distance eso deviation >near eso deviation
        2) Basic eso
           a) Distance eso deviation = near eso deviation
           b) Spasm of the near reflex
           c) Pharmacologic causes (*e.g.,* pilocarpine)

D) Plan
  1) Rx proper refractive correction
  2) Consider plus lens Rx
    a) Determine effectiveness of plus lenses (usually effective due
      to high AC/A ratio)
    b) Repeat near cover test (NCT) with +2.00 D trial frame
    c) Determine AC/A
        1) Example
           a) NCT = 12 Δ esophoria
           b) NCT with +2.00 D Rx = orthophoria
           c) 12 ÷ 2 = 6
           d) AC/A = 6/1
    d) Typical plus Rx = +0.75 D to +1.50 D based on AC/A
        1) If hyperopic refractive error, give plus in addition to
           necessary hyperopia

      2) Consider bifocal Rx if plus lenses decrease distance visual acuity
        a) For school-age children
          1) Flat top option: seg height at lower lid margin
          2) Progressive add lens (PAL): seg height at lower lid margin. Acceptable alternative and typically well tolerated by kids when cosmesis is a concern
3) Consider BO relieving prism (can be used with/without plus lenses)
    a) Rx to achieve Sheard's criteria
      1) Example
        a) Patient findings
          1) Distance cover test = 4 Δ esophoria
          2) Near cover test = 14 Δ intermittent esotropia
          3) Near BI ranges = 18/10 (break/recovery)
        b) Interpretation
          1) Convergence excess
          2) Does not meet Sheard's criteria (2x phoria = break)
            a) To meet Sheard's criteria BI vergence break point (18) would need to be $\geq$ 28 (14 x 2)
          3) Prism Rx of 5 Δ BO (2.5 Δ BO OD, 2.5 Δ BO OS) will allow patient to meet Sheard's criteria
            a) Decreases eso deviation to 9 Δ and allows break point of 18 Δ to meet Sheard's criteria
    b) Full time wear prism Rx if eso deviation exists at distance and near and patient can tolerate without diplopia at distance
    c) Reading only prism Rx if patient has eso deviation at near only
4) Orthoptic training
    a) Vergence training
      1) Concentrate on BI (divergence) skills but be sure to balance with BO (convergence) training
      2) Step I = smooth vergence training
        a) 1st = continuous BI/negative fusional vergence
        b) 2nd = continuous BO/positive fusional vergence
          1) BI prior to BO training because divergence is extremely difficult to achieve after a prolonged convergence trial
        c) Equipment choices
          1) Brock string
          2) Vectograms
          3) Computer orthoptic programs
      3) Step II = jump vergence training
        a) Continuous alternation between BI and BO vergences
        b) Equipment choices
          1) Vectograms
          2) Computer orthoptic programs
      4) Step III = free space circles
        a) Equipment choices

        1) Eccentric circles
        2) Life saver cards
    5) Step IV = integrative techniques (integrating vergence and accommodative skills)
        a) Note: most CE exist with accommodative dysfunction as well. Refer to chapter on diagnosis and treatment of accommodative disorders and incorporate as needed
        b) BO vergence skills with plus lenses (BOP)
        c) BI vergence skills with minus lenses (BIM)
        d) Equipment choices
            1) Vectograms
            2) Flippers of various powers
                a) Begin at +/- 0.50 D, progress to +/- 2.00 D
5) Treatment tips
  a) Plus Rx
    1) Ideal for patients who demonstrate a high AC/A ratio. Typically relieves symptoms and is often the only treatment option necessary
      a) Single vision vs. bifocal
        1) Single vision for patients whose distance VA through Rx = 20/30 or better
        2) Bifocal for patients whose distance VA is reduced and need to alternate fixation from distance ↔ near throughout a day (*e.g.*, school age child, desk jobs, etc.)
    2) Can be used in conjunction with orthoptic program to ease divergence demand
  b) Prism Rx
    1) Ideal for patients who
      a) Demonstrate a residual eso deviation with plus Rx
      b) Have a low AC/A ratio and demonstrate an eso deviation at near as well as distance
  c) Orthoptic training
    1) Lack of success typically coincides with lack of compliance, therefore not an ideal option if patient not committed and/or motivated for orthoptic treatment
  d) Patient examples
    1) Patient 1
      a) 4 Δ esophoria at distance, 10 Δ intermittent esotropia at near
      b) Plus Rx = +1.50 sph OU (PAL)
        1) 20/50 DVA
        2) 3 Δ esophoria (AC/A = 5/1)
      c) Orthoptic program can be added if patient symptoms are not alleviated with plus Rx
    2) Patient 2
      a) 4 Δ esophoria at distance, 16 Δ intermittent esotropia at near

        b) Plus + prism Rx
           1) Plus Rx = +1.50 sph OU (single vision)
              a) 20/30 DVA
              b) 10 Δ esophoria (AC/A = 2/1)
           2) +1.50 OU with 2 Δ BO OD, OS
              a) 6 Δ esophoria remaining and manageable
           3) Orthoptic program can be added if patient symptoms are not alleviated with plus Rx

Notes

29

DIAGNOSIS AND MANAGEMENT OF NEAR POINT BINOCULAR VISION PROBLEMS

CONVERGENCE INSUFFICIENCY (CI)

A) Subjective
    1) Following symptoms associated with near work
        a) Headaches
        b) Asthenopia
        c) Diplopia
        d) Intermittent blur/print moves on page
        e) Fatigue
        f) Avoidance of near tasks
        g) May demonstrate poor reading skills relative to intelligence

B) Objective
    1) Cover test
        a) High exo deviation at near (near >distance)
            1) Normal lateral phoria value = $6 - 8\ \Delta$ exophoria
            2) May break down into intermittent exotropia with fatigue
                and/or prolonged dissociation
    2) NPC
        a) Receded break and recovery in convergence insufficiency
        b) Normal values
            1) Children = break at $6 - 10$ cm
            2) Adults = break at $5 - 7$ cm
        c) Alternative techniques
            1) NPC repeated 5 times to induce fatigue
            2) NPC performed with red lens held over one eye while
                viewing a transilluminator (dissociated effect often creates
                a more receded NPC)
    3) Fusional vergences
        a) Near BO/positive fusional vergences low in convergence
            insufficiency (CI) patients
        b) Near BI/negative fusional vergences normal: high in CI
            patients
        c) Vergence norms

    1) Step/prism bar vergences
      a) Adults (break/recovery)
        1) Near BO = 19/14
        2) Near BI = 13/10
      b) Children 7 – 12 yrs (break/recovery)
        1) Near BO = 23/16
        2) Near BI = 12/7
    2) Smooth/phoropter vergences
      a) All ages (blur/break/recovery)
        1) Near BO = 17/21/11
        2) Near BI = 13/21/13
   d) Compensating vergences based on Sheard's criteria
     1) Break = 2x phoria [see patient example in **D) Plan,** 4)
       Treatment tips below]
  4) Low AC/A ratio
    a) Normal value = 4/1
  5) Stereopsis usually adequate/above adequate with CI
    a) Wirt circles
    b) Random dot
    c) If absent patient may exhibit strabismus/intermittent exotropia
      at near
  6) Accommodative facility testing (using +/- 2.00 D binocular flippers)
    a) Cannot clear plus lenses secondary to poor convergence

C) Assessment
  1) Summary of typical finding
    a) High exo deviation at near
    b) Receded NPC
    c) Low BO vergence ranges
    d) Low AC/A ratio
    e) Adequate stereopsis
    f) Inability to clear plus lenses binocularly
  2) Differential diagnosis
    a) Uncorrected refractive error
    b) Undetected vertical phoria
    c) Other exo classifications
      1) Divergence excess
        a) Distance exo deviation >near exo deviation
      2) Basic exo
        a) Distance exo deviation = near exo deviation
    d) Convergence palsy

D) Plan
  1) Rx proper refractive correction
  2) Consider BI relieving prism
    a) Rx to achieve Sheard's criteria
      1) Example
        a) Patient findings
          1) Distance cover test = 6 Δ exophoria

        2) Near cover test = 12 Δ intermittent exotropia
        3) Near BO (ranges = 16/6 (break/recovery))
    b) Interpretation
        1) Convergence insufficiency
        2) Does not meet Sheard's criteria (phoria = 2x break)
            a) To meet Sheard's criteria, BO vergence break
                point (16 Δ) would need to be $\geq$ 24 (12 x 2)
        3) Prism Rx of 4 Δ BI (2 Δ BI OD, 2 Δ BI OS) will allow
           patient to meet Sheard's criteria
            a) Decreases exo deviation to 8 Δ and allows break
                point of 16 Δ to meet Sheard's criteria
            b) Full time wear prism Rx if exo deviation exists at
                distance and near and patient can tolerate without
                diplopia at distance
            c) Reading only prism Rx if patient has exo deviation
                at near only
3) Orthoptic training
    a) Gross convergence
        1) Pencil push ups
        2) Brock string
    b) Vergence training
        1) Concentrate on BO (convergence) skills, but be sure to
           balance with BI (divergence) training
        2) Step I = smooth vergence training
            a) 1st = continuous BI/negative fusional vergence
            b) 2nd = continuous BO/positive fusional vergence
                 1) BI prior to BO training because divergence is
                   extremely difficult to achieve after a prolonged
                   convergence trial
            c) Equipment choices
                1) Vectograms
                2) Computer orthoptic programs
        3) Step II = jump vergence training
            a) Continuous alternation between BI and BO vergences
            b) Equipment choices
                1) Vectograms
                2) Computer orthoptic programs
        4) Step III = free space circles
            a) Equipment choices
                1) Eccentric circles
                2) Life saver cards
        5) Step IV = integrative techniques (integrating vergence and
           accommodative skills)
            a) Note: most CI exists with accommodative dysfunction
                as well. Refer to chapter on diagnosis and treatment of
                accommodative disorders and incorporate as needed
            b) BO vergence skills with plus lenses (BOP)
            c) BI vergence skills with minus lenses (BIM)

        d) Equipment choices
           1) Vectograms
           2) Flippers of various powers
              a) Begin at +/- 0.50 D, progress to +/- 2.00 D
  4) Treatment tips
    a) Prism Rx
        1) Ideal for patients who demonstrate an exo deviation at near as well as at distance
        2) Can be used in conjunction with orthoptic program to ease convergence demand
        3) Ideal for patients unable to commit to an orthoptic program
    b) Orthoptic training
        1) Excellent treatment option for all convergence insufficiency patients
        2) Lack of success typically coincides with lack of compliance, therefore not an ideal option if patient not committed and/or motivated for orthoptic treatment
    c) Patient examples
        1) Patient 1
           a) 8 Δ exophoria at distance, 16 Δ intermittent exotropia at near
           b) Prism Rx = 3 Δ OD, 3 Δ BI OS
              1) Diplopia not created at near
              2) Patient will now have a more manageable 10 Δ deviation at near and most likely deviate to an exotropia less often
           c) Orthoptic program can be initiated along with prism Rx to improve vergence skills to overcome convergence demand
        2) Patient 2
           a) Orthophoria at distance, 16 Δ intermittent exotropia at near
           b) Prism Rx
              1) Not ideal. If Rxed can typically be used as a reading only. Will create diplopia at distance
              2) Orthoptic training is the best option for this patient

Notes____

30

DIAGNOSIS AND MANAGEMENT OF NEAR POINT BINOCULAR VISION PROBLEMS

ACCOMMODATIVE DYSFUNCTION (AD)

A) Subjective
1) Symptoms associated with near work
- a) Headaches
- b) Asthenopia
- c) Diplopia
- d) Variable visual acuity at distance when looking up from near work
- e) Intermittent blur at near/print moves on page
- f) Fatigue
- g) Avoidance of near tasks
- h) Close working distance
- i) May demonstrate poor reading skills relative to intelligence

B) Objective
1) VA
- a) Fluctuating distance visual acuity
- b) Reduced near visual acuity with minimal refractive error

2) Retinoscopy findings
- a) Pupillary dilation $\rightarrow$ constriction noted
- b) Fluctuating retinoscopy reflex

3) Fusional vergence dysfunction
- a) Often present with accommodative dysfunction (AD)
- b) R/O convergence insufficiency or convergence excess conditions

4) Accommodative tests
- a) Accommodative amplitude measures
    1) Minus lens (preferred method)
    2) Push up/pull away
    3) Normal values = 15 −¼ patient's age
- b) Accommodative facility testing with +/- 2.00 D flippers
    1) CPM = cycles per min

    2) 1 cycle constitutes clearing the plus and the minus side of the flipper
    3) Norms developed for 20/40 print size
      a) Normal values
        1) Binocular testing = 8 cpm
          a) Must monitor for suppression
        2) Monocular testing = 11 cpm
c) MEM
d) NRA/PRA testing [negative (NRA) and positive (PRA) relative accommodation]
    1) Normal values for children and non-presbyopic adults
      a) NRA = +2.50
      b) PRA = - 3.50

C) Assessment
1) Classifications of AD
    a) Accommodative insufficiency
      1) Definition = inability to stimulate accommodation
      2) Objective findings
        a) Amplitudes = decreased
        b) Facility = fails (-) lens binocularly and monocularly
        c) MEM = high lag of accommodation
        d) NRA/PRA = high NRA/low PRA
    b) Accommodative infacility
      1) Definition = poor flexibility of accommodative system. Inability to sustain accommodation
      2) Objective findings
        a) Amplitudes = normal
        b) Facility = fails (-) and (+) lens
        c) MEM = normal, may fluctuate
        d) NRA/PRA = normal or both reduced
    c) Accommodative excess
      1) Definition = inability to relax accommodation
      2) Objective findings
        a) Amplitudes = normal
        b) Facility = fails (+) lens binocularly and monocularly
        c) MEM = lead of accommodation
        d) NRA/PRA = low NRA/high to normal PRA
2) Differential diagnosis
    a) Uncorrected refractive error: perform cycloplegic retinoscopy to R/O hyperopia, pseudomyopia, etc.
    b) Undiagnosed vergence dysfunction with secondary accommodative problem
    c) Spasm of the near reflex
    d) Psychogenic amblyopia
    e) Accommodative paralysis

D) Plan
1) Rx proper refractive correction
2) Consider plus lens Rx for near work
   a) Typical Rx +0.75 D to +1.50 D
   b) Must determine plus acceptance by trial framing desired plus Rx and evaluating
      1) Improvement in near VA
      2) Patient notes print appears larger
      3) Patient reports increased comfort
   c) Must determine effect on distance visual acuity (DVA)
      1) If DVA is reduced, consider Rx in bifocal form
   d) Effect of plus lenses on accommodative dysfunction
      1) Accommodative insufficiency: accepted by most
      2) Accommodative infacility
         a) Accepted by patients with plus acceptance only
         b) Orthoptic training for those who do not accept plus
3) Orthoptic training
   a) Begin with monocular techniques
      1) Minus lens dips
         a) Start at patient's measured amplitude and increase by 1 D each week
         b) Goal = age-appropriate amplitude: 15 −¼ age
         c) Equipment
            1) For in-office procedure may use trial lenses
            2) For home therapy procedure may sell patient appropriate power lens blank
         d) Procedure
            1) Post Hart chart (or any comparable distance letter chart) at 6 ft distance
            2) Patch OS
            3) Dip lens OD, read line 1
            4) Remove lens, read line 2
            5) Complete entire chart
            6) Repeat with other eye
      2) Monocular accommodative facility
         a) Start at a +/- 0.50 D to +/- 1.00 D range
         b) Use 20/40 print
         c) Patient alternates from (+) to (-) lens
         d) Increase by 0.50 D steps weekly or as accepted
         e) Goal: patient achieves task with +/- 2 D
   b) Progress to binocular techniques
      1) Binocular accommodative facility
         a) Start at a +/- 0.50 D to +/- 1.00 D range
         b) Use 20/40 print (monitor for suppression)
         c) Patient alternates from (+) to (-) lens
         d) Increase by 0.50 D steps weekly or as accepted
         e) Goal: patient achieves task with +/- 2 D

Notes

31

DIAGNOSIS AND MANAGEMENT OF NEAR POINT BINOCULAR VISION PROBLEMS

OCULOMOTOR DYSFUNCTION (OMD)

A) Subjective
- 1) Symptoms related to eye movements with reading
    - a) Head movement
    - b) Loses place, skips lines
    - c) Slow reading speed
    - d) Poor reading comprehension
    - e) Following with finger to read

B) Objective
- 1) R/O the following (oculomotor dysfunction (OMD)) rarely exists as a lone diagnosis)
    - a) Uncorrected refractive error
        - 1) Visual acuity
        - 2) Retinoscopy
    - b) Binocular vision anomalies
        - 1) Cover test/phoria measurement
        - 2) Vergences
        - 3) NPC
    - c) Accommodative dysfunction
        - 1) Amplitude measures
        - 2) Facility testing
- 2) Assessment of oculomotor function
    - a) Fixation stability
        - 1) Evaluated during cover test
        - 2) Patient should be capable of maintaining fixation for ~ 10 sec in the absence of noticeable eye movements
    - b) Saccadic/pursuit stability
        - 1) Gross evaluation
            - a) NSUCO oculomotor test (standardized assessment)
                - 1) Set of instructions for observation of patient
                - 2) Set of instructions for appropriate targets
                - 3) Set of instructions for target placement

 4) Set of instructions for scoring system
 5) Normative data provided
2) Measured/objective evaluation
 a) Visagraph II
  1) Infared recording unit used to assess eye movement skills. Printed results generated
   a) Expensive equipment
   b) Patient may be referred for this test
 b) Developmental eye movement test (DEM)
  1) Visual–verbal test of oculomotility
  2) Test eye movements associated with reading
   a) Timed test
   b) Mathematical scoring criteria provided
  3) Aids in differentiating OMD from a visual perceptual disorder
 c) Pursuit skills (isolated)
  1) Southern California College of Optometry (SCCO) test for pursuits
   a) Target size ~ 20/80
   b) Test distance = 40 cm
   c) Move target in horizontal/vertical/diagonal directions
   d) Scoring system
    1) 4+ = smooth and accurate pursuits
    2) 3+ = 1 fixation loss
    3) 2+ = 2 fixation losses
    4) 1+ = more than 2 fixation losses
     a) A score of less than 3+ indicates a pursuit problem
 d) Saccadic skills (isolated)
  1) SCCO test for saccades
   a) Target size ~ 20/80
   b) Test distance = 40 cm
   c) 2 targets spaced 25 cm apart
   d) Examiner instructs patient to look from one target to the other about 10 times
   e) Scoring system
    1) 4+ = smooth and accurate saccades
    2) 3+ = slight undershoot
    3) 2+ = gross undershoot or overshoot
    4) 1+ = inability to perform task
    a) A score of less than 3+ indicates a saccadic problem

C) Assessment
1) Differential diagnosis
 a) Uncorrected refractive error
 b) Neurologic disease/gaze disturbance

    c) Binocular vision/accommodative dysfunction
    d) Common side effects of medication

D) Plan
    1) Rx proper refractive correction
    2) Orthoptic training
        a) Typical treatment time = 8 – 24 sessions
        b) Home therapy activities prescribed daily = 20 min/day
        c) Goal attained when subjective complaints and objective test findings have improved
            1) Gross activities
                a) Hart chart saccades
                b) Groffman tracings
                c) Wayne saccadic fixator
                d) Mazes/dot to dot
                e) Marsden ball
            2) Computer orthopter activities
                a) Pursuits
                b) Saccades
                c) Tachistoscope
                d) Word/letter searches
            3) Integration of oculomotor function with vergence and accommodative skill

Notes
____

APPENDIX

COLOR CODING FOR RETINAL DRAWING

A) Black
   1) Basic sketch outlines
   2) Borders
   3) Pigment
   4) Nevi

B) Brown
   1) Choroidal detachments
   2) Choroidal melanoma
   3) Choroidal neovascular membrane
   4) Drusen

C) Blue
   1) Detached retina
   2) Subsensory or subretinal fluid or retinal edema
   3) Cotton wool patches
   4) Inner layer of retinoschisis
   5) Rolled edges of retinal tears and breaks
   6) Area of detached retina
   7) Detached macula, drawn as a blue cross
   8) Traction tufts or cysts
   9) Retinal veins

D) Green
   1) Epiretinal membrane
   2) Retinal operculum
   3) Vitreous hemorrhage
   4) Asteroid bodies
   5) Intra-ocular foreign body
   6) Fibrous proliferation

E) Red
   1) Open area of retinal holes or tears
   2) Intra-retinal hemorrhages
   3) Pre-retinal hemorrhages, background retinopathy
   4) Attached area of retina
   5) Normal fovea, drawn as a red cross
   6) Retinal collateral or shunt vessels

F) Yellow
   1) Intra-retinal or sub-retinal exudates
   2) Detached macula from serous or hemorrhage, drawn as a yellow
      cross

G) Orange
   1) Elevated retinal neovascularization of the disk or elsewhere

H) Purple
   1) Flat retinal neovascularization of the disk or elsewhere

EYECARE ABBREVIATIONS

Δ	prism diopters
A&O×3	alert and oriented to person, place and time
A/V	arterial/venous ratio
AACG	acute angle closure glaucoma
ABK	aphakic bullous keratopathy
ac	ante cibum (before meals)
AC	anterior chamber
AC/A	accommodative convergence/accommodation ratio
Acc	accommodation
ACE	angiotensin converting enzyme
ACG	angle closure glaucoma
AD	accommodative dysfunction
ad lib	at discretion
Add	adduction
ADHD	attention deficit hyperactivity disorder
ADR	adverse drug reaction
AIDS	acquired immunodeficiency syndrome
AION	anterior ischemic optic neuropathy
ALT	argon laser trabeculoplasty
AMA	against medical advice
Amb	ambulatory
AMPPPE	acute multifocal posterior placoid pigment epitheliopathy
ANA	antinuclear antibodies
ANCA	anti-neutrophil cytoplasmic antibody
APD	afferent pupillary defect
AR	Argyll Robertson, auto refraction
ARC	anomalous retinal correspondence
ARG	angle recession glaucoma
ARMD	age related macular degeneration
ARN	acute retinal necrosis
ASA	acetylsalicylic acid
ATR	against the rule astigmatism
BAT	brightness acuity testing
BC	base curve
BCP	birth control pill
BD	base down
BDR	background diabetic retinopathy (use non-proliferative diabetic retinopathy instead)
BI	base in prism
bid	twice per day
BIO	binocular indirect ophthalmoscopy

BO	base out prism
bleph	blepharitis
BP	blood pressure
BRAO	branch retinal artery occlusion
BRVO	branch retinal vein occlusion
BS	blood sugar
BU	base up prism
BUN	blood urea nitrogen
BVP	back vertex power
Bx	biopsy
C	cornea
C & S	culture and sensitivity
C/O	complains of
CA	cancer
CACG	chronic angle closure glaucoma
CAI	carbonic anhydrase inhibitor
CAT	computerized axial tomography
cat	cataract
CB	color blind, caesarian birth
CBC	complete blood count
CC	chief complaint, cum (with) correction
CD	cup to disk ratio
CF	count fingers, confrontation field
CHA	compound hyperopic astigmatism
CHF	congestive heart failure
CI	convergence insufficiency
cl	clear
CL	contact lens
CLARE	contact lens associated red eye
CMA	compound myopic astigmatism
CME	cystoid macular edema
CMV	cytomegalovirus
CNVM	choroidal neovascular membrane
COAG	chronic open angle glaucoma
COPD	chronic obstructive pulmonary disease
CP	cerebral palsy
CRAO	central retinal artery occlusion
CRVO	central retinal vein occlusion
CSDME	clinically significant diabetic macular edema
CSF	cerebrospinal fluid
CSME	clinically significant macular edema
CT	computerized tomography, cover test
CV	color vision
CVA	cerebrovascular accident

CWS	cotton wool spot
D	diopters
D & I	dilation and irrigation
D & Q	deep and quiet
D/C	discontinue
D-C	dermatochalasis
db	decibel
DCR	dacryocystorhinostomy
DD	disk diameter
DDx	differential diagnosis
DFE	dilated fundus examination
Dk	oxygen permeability
Dk/L	oxygen transmissibility
DM	diabetes mellitus
DOB	date of birth
DOE	dyspnea on exertion
DW	daily wear
Dx	diagnosis
EBMD	epithelial basement membrane disease
ECCE	extracapsular cataract extraction
ECG	electrocardiogram
EEG	electroencephalogram
EKC	epidemic keratoconjunctivitis
EKG	electrocardiogram
E/M	evaluation and management coding
EOG	electrooculogram
EOM	extra ocular muscles
EP	esophoria
ERG	electroretinography
ERM	epiretinal membrane
ESR	erythrocyte sedimentation rate
ET	esotropia
EW	extended wear
F/U	Follow-up
FA	fluorescein angiogram
FANG	fluorescein angiogram
FAZ	foveal avascular zone
FB	foreign body
FBS	fasting blood sugar
FDT	frequency doubling technology
FESA	full equal smooth accurate
FHN	family history negative
FHP	family history positive
GCA	giant cell arteritis

gtt	drops
H	hyperopia
H & E	hemorrhage and exudation
H/O	history of
HA	headache
Hb	hemoglobin
HbA1c	glycosylated hemoglobin
HCTZ	hydrochlorothiazide
HDL	high density lipoproteins
HHP	Hollenhorst plaque
HIV	human immunodeficiency virus
HLA	human leukocyte antigens
HM	hand motion
HPI	history of present illness
HPPM	hyperplastic persistent pupillary membrane
HR	heart rate
hs	at bedtime
HSV	herpes simplex virus
HTN	hypertension
Hx	history
HZV	herpes zoster virus
I	iris
ICCE	intra capsular cataract extraction
ICG	indocyanine green
ICP	intra cranial pressure
IDDM	insulin dependent diabetes mellitus
IM	intramuscular
Inf	infection
inj	injection
IO	intraocular
IOL	intraocular lens
IOP	intraocular pressure
IRMA	intraretinal microvascular abnormalities
IV	intravenous
J	Jaeger test type
JRA	juvenile rheumatoid arthritis
K	keratometry
KDA	known drug allergy
KP	keratitic precipitates
L	lens
LAS	left arm sitting (BP measure)
LASIK	laser intrastromal keratomileusis
LBP	lower back pain
LBW	low birth weight

LDL	low density lipoproteins
LE	left eye
LL	lower lid
LLL	left lower lid
LME	last medical exam
LP	lumbar puncture
LP	light perception
LPI	laser peripheral iridectomy
LTG	low tension glaucoma
LUL	left upper lid
m	meter
M	myopia
M&N	Mydriacyl and Neo-Synepherine
MA	mental age, mixed astigmatism
ME	macular edema
MEM	monocular estimation method
MEWDS	multifocal evanescent white dot syndrome
MG	myasthenia gravis, Marcus Gunn
MGD	meibomian gland disease
MI	myocardial infarction
MR	manifest refraction
MRI	magnetic resonance imaging
MS	multiple sclerosis
MVA	motor vehicle accident
N & V	nausea and vomiting
NA	not applicable
NAION	non-arteritic anterior ischemic optic neuropathy
NC	no change
NCT	non-contact tonometry
Nd:YAG	Neodymium: yttrium-aluminum-garnet
neg	negative
neo	neovascularization
NFL	nerve fiber layer
NIDDM	non-insulin dependent diabetes
NKA	no known allergies
NKDA	no known drug allergies
NLP	no light perception
NPC	near point of convergence
NPO	nothing by mouth
NRA	negative relative accommodation
NRC	normal retinal correspondence
NS	no show for appointment
NS	nuclear sclerosis
NSAID	non-steroidal anti-inflammatory drug

NVD	neovascularization of the disk
NVE	neovascularization elsewhere
NVI	neovascularization of the iris
NVG	neovascular glaucoma
OD	oculus dexter (right eye)
OGTT	oral glucose tolerance test
OKN	optokinetic nystagmus
OMD	oculomotor dysfunction
ONH	optic nerve head
OS	oculus sinister (left eye)
OTC	over-the-counter
OU	oculus uterque (both eyes)
PAL	progressive add lens
PAM	potential acuity meter
PAN	preauricular node
PAS	peripheral anterior synechiae
PBK	pseudophakic bullous keratopathy
PC	posterior chamber
PCIOL	posterior chamber intraocular lens
PD	interpupillary distance or prism diopter
PDR	proliferative diabetic retinopathy
PEE	punctate epithelial erosions
PEK	punctate epithelial keratitis
PERRLA	pupils equal, round, responsive to light, accommodation
PET	positron emission tomography
Pg	pregnant
PG	previous glasses
PGF	paternal grandfather
PGM	paternal grandmother
PH	pinhole, personal history
PH NI	pinhole no improvement
PHx	personal history
PI	peripheral iridectomy
PK	penetrating keratoplasty
PLT	preferential looking technique
PMFSH	personal, medical, family and social history
PMHx	personal medical history
PMMA	polymethyl methacrylate
PO	per os (by mouth)
POAG	primary open angle glaucoma
POH	presumed ocular histoplasmosis
POHx	personal ocular history
PP	punctal plug or pressure patch

PPBS	postprandial blood sugar
PPD	purified protein derivative
PPDR	preproliferative diabetic retinopathy
PPM	persistent pupillary membrane
PPV	pars plana vitrectomy
PRA	positive relative accommodation
PRH	preretinal hemorrhage
PRK	photorefractive keratectomy
prn	as needed
PS	posterior synechiae
PSC	posterior subcapsular cataract
PTC	pseudotumor cerebri
PTK	photo therapeutic keratectomy
PUD	peptic ulcer disease
PVD	posterior vitreous detachment
PVR	proliferative vitreoretinopathy
PXG	pseudoexfoliation glaucoma
PXS	pseudoexfoliation syndrome
qd	once per day
qhs	every evening
qid	four times per day
qod	every other day
R	respiration or rate
R/O	rule out
RA	rheumatoid arthritis
RAPD	relative afferent pupillary defect
RAS	right arm sitting (BP measure)
RCE	recurrent corneal erosion
RD	retinal detachment
REM	rapid eye movement
RET	retinoscopy
RF	rheumatoid factor
R-G	red green
RGP	rigid gas permeable
RH	retinal hemorrhage
RHS	right-hand side
RK	radial keratotomy
RLF	retrolental fibroplasia
RLL	right lower lid
ROP	retinopathy of prematurity
ROS	review of systems
RP	retinitis pigmentosa
RPE	retinal pigment epithelium
RPR	rapid plasma reagin

RR	respiratory rate
RSM	relative spectacle magnification
RTC	return to clinic
RUL	right upper lid
Rx	prescribe
S/P	status post
SAFE	smooth accurate full and equal
sc	sans (without) correction
SCAN	suspected child abuse and neglect
SCH	sub conjunctival heme
SCL	soft contact lens
sed rate	erythrocyte sedimentation rate
SEI	sub epithelial infiltrate
SL	slit lamp, Schwalbe's line
SLACH	soft lens associated chronic hypoxia
SLE	systemic lupus erythematosus
SLK	superior limbic keratoconjunctivitis
SO	superior oblique
SOAP	subjective, objective, assessment, plan
SOB	shortness of breath
SR	superior rectus
SRF	subretinal fluid
SRH	subretinal hemorrhage
SS	scleral spur, Sjögren's syndrome
sol	solution
Sph	spherical
SPK	superficial punctate keratitis
SRNVM	subretinal neovascular membrane
SSF	sub-sensory fluid
stat	immediately
STD	sexually transmitted disease
susp	suspension
SVP	spontaneous venous pulsation
Sx	symptoms
T3	triiodothyronine
T4	thyroxine
TA	tonometry applanation or temporal arteritis
tab	tablet
TB	tuberculosis
TBUT	tear break up time
TED	thyroid eye disease
TIA	transient ischemic attack
tid	three times per day
TM	trabecular meshwork

TNTC	too numerous to count
TP	Tono Pen
TPR	temperature, pulse, respiration
Trig	triglycerides
TVL	transient vision loss
UBM	ultrasound biomicroscope
ud	ut dictum (as directed)
UGH	uveitis, glaucoma, hyphema
UL	upper lid
ung	ointment
URI	upper respiratory infection
US	ultrasonography
UTI	urinary tract infection
UV	ultraviolet
VA	visual acuity
VAcc	visual acuity with correction
VAsc	visual acuity without correction
VDRL	Venereal Disease Research Laboratory
VEP	visual evoked potential
VF	visual field
VG	von Graefe phorias
VKC	vernal keratoconjunctivitis
VLDL	very low density lipoproteins
VM	visual memory
VS	vital signs
VSR	venous stasis retinopathy
W4D	Worth 4 Dot
WBC	white blood cells
WCB	wheelchair bound
w	with
wk	week
wo	with out
WNL	within normal limits
WPOA	wearing patch on arrival
WTR	with the rule astigmatism
XO	exophthalmos
XP	exophoria
XR	x-ray
XT	exotropia
YAG	yttrium aluminum garnet
Y-B	yellow-blue color defect
yo	yrs old
⊖	negative
⊕	positive

VISION STANDARDS

A) Driver's license visual acuity standards
1) Washington DC: 20/40 in one eye, and 20/70 in the other
2) West Virginia: 20/60 in either eye
3) All other states: 20/40 in either eye
4) Bioptic device permitted: Alaska, Arkansas, California, Colorado, Delaware, DC, Georgia, Hawaii, Idaho, Illinois, Indiana, Iowa, Kansas, Louisiana, Maryland, Massachusetts, Michigan, Missouri, Montana, Nebraska, Nevada, New Hampshire, New Jersey, New York, Ohio, South Dakota, Texas, Vermont, Virginia, Wisconsin, Wyoming
5) Telescopic device permitted: Alaska, Arkansas, California, Colorado, Delaware, DC, Idaho, Illinois, Indiana, Kansas, Maryland, Massachusetts, Missouri, Montana, Nebraska, Nevada, New Hampshire, New Jersey, New York, North Dakota, Ohio, South Dakota, Tennessee, Texas, Vermont, Washington, Wyoming

B) Commercial driver's license standards: see following table

C) Sport pilot: valid driver's license

D) Third class medical (private pilot)
1) Uncorrected distance VA: no minimum
2) Corrected distance VA: 20/40 in each eye, correctable by glasses or contacts, or refractive surgery
3) Near VA: 20/40 at 16 inches in each eye with or without lenses
4) Monovision is not allowed
5) No acute or chronic pathology that interferes with function or may be reasonably expected to be aggravated by flying
6) Color vision
   a) 14 plate Ishihara: <6 errors on plates 1 – 11
   b) 24 plate Ishihara: <7 errors on plates 1 – 15
   c) 38 plate Ishihara: <9 errors on plates 1 – 21
   d) AO color test: <7 errors on plates 1 – 15
7) Waivers: a Statement of Demonstrated Ability may be issued to applicants who do not meet these standards if the disqualifying condition is non-progressive and they have been found capable of performing airman duties without endangering public safety
8) Duration of certificate: if younger than 40 yrs old, certificate is good for 36 months after the end of the month of examination. If 40 or older, certificate is good for 24 months after the end of the month of examination

VISION STANDARDS FOR COMMERCIAL DRIVERS

	VISUAL ACUITY BINOC	VISUAL FIELD MONOC	BINOC	COLOR	OTHER	RETEST
Alabama	20/70	No	No	No	No	No
Alaska	20/40	No	No	No	No	Periodic
Arizona	20/40	No	No	No	No	Periodic
Arkansas	20/50	NS	NS	NS	NS	NS
California	20/40	70, 70	NS	R,G,A	NS	Periodic
Colorado	20/40	Yes	Yes	Yes	ST	Periodic
Connecticut	20/40	Yes	Yes	Yes	ST	No
Delaware	20/40	No	No	No	No	Periodic
Florida	20/70	No	No	No	No	Periodic
Georgia	20/60	140, 140	140	No	No	Periodic
Hawaii	20/40	70, 70	140	R,G,A	ST, EC	Periodic
Idaho	20/40	NS	NS	NS	NS	Periodic
Illinois	20/40	70, 70	140	NS	NS	Periodic
Indiana	20/50	No	No	No	NS	Periodic
Iowa	20/70	No	No	No	NS	Periodic
Kansas	20/40	NS	NS	NS	NS	Periodic
Kentucky	20/45, PV	No	No	No	No	No
Louisiana	20/40	No	No	No	No	Periodic
Maine	20/40	NS	NS	NS	NS	No
Maryland	20/40	140, 140	140	No	No	Periodic
Massachusetts	20/40	90, 90	120	Yes	No	Periodic
Michigan	20/40	70, 70	140	NS	NS	Periodic
Minnesota	20/40	NS	NS	NS	NS	Periodic
Mississippi	20/40	90, 90	180	No	ST	No
Missouri	20/40	55, 55	No	No	No	Periodic
Montana	20/40	75, 75	No	Yes	ST	Periodic
Nebraska	20/40	70, 70	140	Yes	No	Periodic
Nevada	20/40	No	No	No	No	Periodic
New Hamshire	20/40	NS	NS	NS	NS	Periodic
New Jersey	20/40	70, 70	No	R,G,A	No	NS
New Mexico	20/40	NS	NS	NS	NS	Periodic
New York	20/40	NS	NS	NS	NS	Periodic
North Carolina	20/50	No	70	Yes	No	Periodic
North Dacota	20/40	70, 70	140	No	No	Periodic
Ohio	20/40	70, 70	No	No	No	Periodic
Oklahoma	20/40	No	No	No	No	No
Oregon	20/40	No	110	No	No	No
Pennsylvania	20/40	No	140	No	No	No
Rhode Island	20/40	60, 60	120	Yes	No	Periodic
South Carolina	PV	NS	NS	NS	NS	Periodic
South Dakota	20/40	No	No	No	No	Periodic
Tennessee	20/40	No	No	No	No	No
Texas	20/50	No	No	No	No	Periodic
Utah	20/40	NS	NS	Yes	ST	Periodic
Vermont	20/40	NS	NS	NS	NS	No
Verginia	20/40	100, 100	100	No	NS	Periodic
Washington	20/40	No	140	R,G,A	No	Periodic
West Virginia	20/40	No	No	No	No	No
Wisconsin	20/40	70, 70	140	No	No	Periodic
Wyoming	20/40	No	No	No	No	Periodic

Key: Visual acuity is expressed in Snellen notation; visual field is given in degree along the horizontal meridian; color abbreviati-ons: R = red, G = green, A = amber; abbreviations for other conditions: EC = eye coordinations; ST = stereopsis (absence of); NS = standard no specified; No = no standard; PV = default to private vehicle standard.

Source: US Dept of Transportation. *Visual Disorders and Commercial Drivers*. Washington, DC: Federal Highway Administra-tion, Office of Motor Carriers; Nov 1991. US Dept of Transportation publication FHWA-MC-92-003, HCS-10/1-92(200)E.

E) Second class medical (commercial pilot): all of the above plus the following requirements
1) Corrected distance VA 20/20 in each eye, corrected by glasses, contacts or refractive surgery
2) Intermediate VA if 50 or older: 20/40 at 32 inches with or without lenses
3) Hyperphoria: 1 Δ maximum
4) Lateral phoria: 6 Δ eso or exophoria
5) Field of vision: normal fields of vision (as measured grossly)
6) Duration of certificate: 12 months after the end of the month of examination

F) First class medical (airline pilot): same requirements as second class
1) Duration of certificate: 6 months after the end of the month of examination

G) US Coast Guard Academy: these are the most common requirements; they are not all-inclusive
1) Uncorrected VA of 20/400 in each eye
2) Correctable to 20/20 in each eye for distance
3) Correctable to 20/60 in best eye for near
4) Refractive error not more than + or −6.00 D in any meridian
5) Astigmatism not >3.00 D
6) Anisometropia not >3.50 D
7) Normal binocularity
8) Normal motility
9) Normal color vision
10) Standards for refractive surgery are in flux. If prohibited, have the applicant inquire about a waiver

H) US Merchant Marine Academy: these are the most common requirements; they are not all-inclusive
1) Uncorrected VA of 20/400 in each eye
2) Correctable to 20/20 in each eye at distance
3) Correctable to 20/60 at near in the best eye
4) Refractive error not more than + or −6.00 D in any meridian
5) Astigmatism not >3.00 D
6) Anisometropia not >3.50 D
7) Normal binocularity
8) Normal motility
9) Normal color vision
10) Standards for refractive surgery are in flux. If prohibited, have the applicant inquire about a waiver

I) US Naval Academy: these are the most common requirements, they are not all-inclusive
1) Uncorrected distance VA of 20/20 in each eye

2) Waivers may be given if correctable to 20/20 in each eye and within certain refractive standards
    a) Refractive error not more than + or −6.00 D in any meridian
    b) Astigmatism not >3.00 D
    c) Anisometropia not >3.50 D
3) Normal binocularity
4) Normal motility
5) Normal color vision
6) Standards for refractive surgery are in flux. Even if prohibited, have the applicant inquire about a waiver

J) US Military Academy: these are the most common requirements, they are not all-inclusive
1) Distance VA correctable to 20/20 in each eye
2) Refractive error not more than + or −8.00 spherical equivalent
3) Astigmatism not >3.00 D
4) Color vision: able to distinguish vivid red and green
5) Esotropia not more than 15 Δ
6) Exotropia not more than 10 Δ
7) Hypertropia less than 5 Δ
8) Normal motility
9) Standards for refractive surgery are in flux. A Department of Defense medical panel recently concluded that refractive surgery does not adversely affect the structure of the eye. It could actually improve soldiers' performance by eliminating hazards associated with eye glasses and contact lenses in combat

K) US Air Force Academy: these are the most common requirements; they are not all-inclusive. Standards for refractive surgery are in flux. If prohibited, have the applicant inquire about a waiver
1) Pilots
    a) Uncorrected distance VA 20/50 in each eye
    b) Distance VA correctable to 20/20 in each eye
    c) Uncorrected near VA 20/20 in each eye
    d) Hyperopia no more than +2.00 D in any meridian
    e) No more than −1.00 myopia in any meridian
    f) Astigmatism no more than 0.75 D
    g) Anisometropia no more than 2.00 D
    h) Normal color vision
    i) Normal depth perception
    j) Normal binocularity
    k) Normal motility
2) Navigator
    a) Uncorrected distance VA 20/200 in each eye
    b) Distance VA correctable to 20/20 in each eye
    c) Near corrected VA 20/20 in each eye
    d) Myopia no more than −2.25 D in any meridian

       e) Hyperopia no more than +3.00 D
       f) Astigmatism no more than 2.00 D
       g) Anisometropia no more than 2.50 D
       h) Normal color vision
       i) Normal binocularity
       j) Normal motility
       k) Normal depth perception
   3) Commissioned officer
       a) Distance VA correctable to 20/40 in one eye and 20/70 in the other, or 20/30 in one eye and 20/100 in the other, or 20/400 in one eye and 20/20 in the other
       b) Near corrected VA 20/40 or better in best eye
       c) Refractive error not more than + or −8.00 D spherical equivalent
       d) Normal binocularity
       e) Normal motility

L) General Department of Defense vision requirements for other military applicants who are not going to a service academy. Many specialties such as pilots and Special Forces are more restrictive
   1) Distance VA correctable to 20/40 in better eye and 20/70 in worse eye
   2) Distance VA correctable to 20/30 in better eye and 20/100 in worse eye
   3) Distance VA correctable to 20/20 in better eye and 20/400 in worse eye
   4) Near VA 20/40 in the better eye
   5) Refraction + or −8.00 D spherical equivalent
   6) No eyeglass problems such as ghost images or prismatic displacement issues
   7) No orthokeratology correction
   8) No medically necessary contacts such as for corneal scarring or irregular astigmatism
   9) Color standards by individual services
   10) Visual fields in degrees
       a) Temporal 85
       b) Superior temporal 55
       c) Superior 45
       d) Superior nasal 55
       e) Nasal 60
       f) Inferior nasal 50
       g) Inferior 65
       h) Inferior temporal 85
   11) No strabismus if uncorrectable by lenses to less than 40 D, or accompanied by diplopia, or corrective surgery in the preceding 6 months. Additional requirements are set by individual services
   12) No eye diseases or degenerations are allowed except for
       a) Blepharitis, if mild only

      b) Pterygium if less than 3 mm encroachment on the cornea, is non-progressive, and non-recurrent

      c) Corneal vascularization if non-progressive and does not reduce vision below the listed vision standards

      d) A single episode of healed chorioretinitis that has healed and does not interfere with vision

13) No history of refractive surgery, though waivers are usually granted for PRK and LASIK 6 months after surgery with full documentation of all exams and post-op reports

Notes for all service academies

1) Do not attempt to "fudge" results when reporting to the Department of Defense. If the military reviewers find the candidate's vision does not meet their standards, the candidate will be rejected later anyway. The candidate will miss the chance to get into another college

2) All services disqualify any applicant who has had refractive surgery, **but** they also usually grant waivers for PRK and LASIK if the pre-operative refraction meets the listed standards

3) Certain specialties such as Special Forces waiver, only PRK

4) Only PRK and LASIK are waivered, not RK or anything else

5) Post-op BCVA must meet standards listed

6) The Air Force requires a 12 month wait since the last surgery or enhancement. The other services require a 6 month wait

7) The post-op refraction must be stable with no significant side effects

8) There must be no lattice or other pathology associated with myopia or hyperopia

9) The complete medical history, copies of all examinations and operative reports are reviewed

10) Standards for refractive surgery are in flux: always have the applicant inquire about a waiver if he/she has had PRK or LASIK

Diagnosis Codes

Symptom codes

Asthenopia	368.13
Blurry vision	368.8
Diplopia	368.2
Dizziness	780.4
Epiphoria	375.20
Floaters	379.24
Headache NOS	784.0
Headache, migraine	346.9
Pain in/around eye	379.91
Photophobia	368.13
Red eye	379.93
Visual disturbance	368.9

Refractive Errors

Astigmatism	367.20
Hyperopia	367.0
Myopia	367.1
Presbyopia	367.4

Vision/Binoc.

Acc. paresis	367.51
Acc. spasm	367.53
Amblyopia, NOS	368.00
Conv. excess	378.84
Conv. insufficiency	378.83
Esotropia, NOS	378.00
Exotropia, monoc.	378.01
Nystagmus NOS	379.50
Phoria	378.40
Saccadic deficiency	379.57
Supression	368.31
Sixth nerve palsy	378.54
Version deficiency	379.58

Lids/ Lac./Orbit

Black eye, NOS	921.0
Bleph, squamous	373.0
Chalazion	373.2
Contusion, ocular	921.1
Dermatochalasis	374.87
Dry eye syndrome	375.15
Ectropion, eyelid	374.10
Entropion, Invol.	374.00
Hordeolum	373.11
Meibomianitis	373.12
Myokymia	307.20
Ptosis NOS	374.30
Trichiasis	374.05
Viral Warts	078.10

Conj. / Sclera

Blepharoconj, NOS	372.20
Conj, allergic, acute	372.00
Conj, allergic, chronic	372.10
Conj, simple, chronic	372.11
Conj, viral, NOS	077.99
Episcleritis, nodular	379.02
FB, conjunctiva	930.1
Heme, subconj	372.72
Pinguecula	372.51
Pterygium, NOS	372.40

Cornea

Abrasion	918.1
Arcus Senilus	371.41
EBMD	371.50
Edema, NOS	371.20
Erosion	371.42
Foreign body	930.0
Fuchs endo. dyst.	371.57
Kerataconus	371.60
Keratitis, punctate	370.21
Neovascularization	370.60
Opacity, central	371.03
Opacity, peripheral	371.02
Ulcer, marginal	370.01
Ulcer, central	370.03

Glaucoma

Angle closure, acute	365.22
Angle close, chronic	365.23
C/D large, physiolo.	**365**
Low tension	**365.12**
Ocular hypertension	365.04
Pigmentary	365.13
Primary open angle	**365.11**
Suspect, borderline	365.00
High Risk Pat, screen	V80.1

Anterior Chamber

Angle recession	364.77
Synechia, Posterior	364.71
Uveitis, primary	364.01
Uveitis, chronic	364.10

Lens

Cortical cataract	366.2
Diabetic cataract	366.41
Nuclear cataract	366.04
Post. subcaps. cat	366.02
Aphakia	379.31
Pseudoexfoliation	366.11
Pseudophakia	V43.1
Second. cat, VA ok	366.52
Second. cat, blurred	366.53

Vitreous

Asteroid hyalitis	379.22
Degen or Detach	379.21
Hemorrhage	379.23

Retina

ARMD, dry	**362.51**
ARMD, exudative	**362.52**
Artheritis (Plaquenil)	714.0
BRVO	362.4
CRVO	362.4
Central serous	362.41
Chorioretinal scar	363.30
CNVM	362.16
Cystoid mac. edema	362.53
Diabetes w/o manifest	250.00
Diabetes, B/R ret	**362.01**
Diabetes, prolif. ret	**362.02**
Diabetic mac. Edema	362.07
Epiretinal membrane	362.56
Hemorrhage, retinal	362.81
High Blood Glucose	790.29
Hypertension, (by hx)	401.9
Hypertensive ret.	362.11
Lattice degeneration	362.63
Macular scar	363.32
Myopic retinal degen	360.60
Nevus, choroidal	224.6
Pavingstone degen.	362.61
Reticular degen.	362.64
Retinal detachment	361.9
Retinal tear	361.30
Retinal hole	361.31

Optic Nerve

Benign Cranial Htn.	377.00
Choloboma	377.23
Drusen	377.21
Ischemic optic neuro.	377.41
Optic atrophy, primary	377.11
Optic nerve hypoplasia	377.43
Optic neuritis	377.30
Retrobulbar neuritis	377.32
Giant Cell arteritis	446.5

Visual Field Defects

Arcuate defects	368.43
General constriction	368.45
Other VF defect	368.40
TIA	435.9

Bold codes require pqri coding

EXAMPLES OF COMMON EYECARE PROCEDURE CODES WITH YEAR 2008 MEDICARE ALLOWABLES FOR NEBRASKA

VISION EXAM CODES	CODE	Medicare Allow
Comp vision exam new	92004	$116.22
Comp vision exam established	92014	$94.70
Int vision exam new	92002	$61.40
Int vision exam established	92012	$65.04
MEDICAL OFFICE CALL CODES		
Comp medical exam new	99205	$162.32
Comp medical exam established	99215	$113.43
Int medical exam new	99204	$128.95
Int medical exam established	99214	$83.87
Lim medical exam new	99203	$83.75
Lim medical exam established	99213	$55.77
Brief medical exam new	99202	$57.19
Brief medical exam established	99212	$34.11
Minimal medical exam established (dcl check)	99211	$17.94
OTHER		
Refraction, <= age 18, brief only	92015	$0.00
Refraction Intermediate or Adult	92015	$0.00
Refraction extended or cycloplegic	92015	$0.00
CL exam surcharge, waived if compliant	92314	$0.00
After hours	99050	$0.00
After hours (10pm – 8am)	99052	$0.00
Glaucoma Screening for high risk patients	G0117	$40.22
PROCEDURES		
Bandage contact lens, fit and supply	92070	$57.13
Cilia epilation	67820	$41.99
Color vision testing, extended	92283	$36.55
Cornea debridement	65435	$62.62
Cornea scrape for culture	65430	$90.03
Dilate w/ or w/o irrigate lacrimal duct	68810	$181.96
FB removal eyelid	67938	$200.97
FB removal conjunctival embedded	65210	$54.24
FB removal corneal embedded	65222	$59.64
FB Rust ring removal	65435	$62.62
GDX per eye (pc $16.57, tc $21.75)	92135	$38.61
Gonioscopy	92020	$22.44
Lid abscess drainage	67700	$220.68
Low vision analysis, telescope	92354	$0.00
Ophthalmoscopy, extended, **per eye**	92225	$20.43
Ophthalmoscopy, subsequent, **per eye**	92226	$18.57

Pachymetry (pc $8.20, tc $2.82)	76514	$11.01
Photos, external series (pc $27.54, tc $9.67)	92285	$37.02
Photos, fundus series (pc $43.33, tc $21.30)	92250	$62.48
Provocative glaucoma test	92140	$48.47
Punctal plug insert-bilat. 1st pr. 10-day post op	68761-50	$174.18
Punctal plug insert-bilat. 2nd pr. 10-day post op	68761-50	$87.09
Sensorimotor exam (pc $39.06, tc$9.76)	92060	$48.82
Serial tonometry	92100	$74.45
Special report	99080	$0.00
Sterile tray	99070	$0.00
Tear quantification	92499	$0.00
Visual Fields Intermediate(pc $37.42, tc $20.36)	92082	$57.78
Visual Fields Threshold (pc $43.13, tc $23.27)	92083	$66.40
Wart destruction first lesion, 10 day post op	17000	$91.98
Wart destruction, 2nd & 3rd lesion, each	17003	$41.30

Consultations, new (with request from provider)

Comprehensive	99245	$205.46
Intermediate	99244	$166.57
Limited	99243	$112.63
Brief	99242	$81.86
Minimal	99241	$43.82

Post op surgery

ALT post op (90-day period)	65855-55	$52.83
Cataract post-op (90-day period)	66984-55	$117.06
Peripheral iridectomy (90-day period)	66761-55	$68.88
Refractive surgery post op per eye		$0.00
YAG post-op (90-day period)	66821-55	$49.13

Other E & M codes	**CODE**	**Med**
Consults, new or established, out-patient	99241	$43.82
	99242	$81.86
	99243	$112.63
	99244	$166.57
	99245	$205.46
Inpatient hospital care, new or established	99234	$115.29
	99235	$152.31
	99236	$189.67
E&M nursing home new	99304	$72.54
	99305	101.08
	99306	129.61
E&M nursing home established	99307	$35.65

	99308	$54.83
	99309	$73.08
	99310	$107.44
E&M home services new	99341	$49.67
	99342	$72.78
	99343	$115.81
	99344	$151.82
	99345	$182.55
E&M home services established	99347	$47.82
	99348	$72.12
	99349	$105.46
	99350	$147.72

Explanation of Medicare Modifiers

LT Left eye
QB Used for the physician shortage area bonus, if you practice in one of these areas
RT Right eye
TC Technical component: used when fields or photos are split into 80% professional and 20% technical charges
21 Prolonged E&M Services: When face to face time provided is greater than usually required for the highest level of E&M services. A report may be necessary
22 Unusual Procedures Services: When the service is greater than that usually required for the listed procedure. A report may be necessary
24 For unrelated evaluation and management service by the same physician during a post-operative period
25 Used when billing for a separately identifiable service the same day as a surgical procedure code (6000 series), by the same physician
26 Professional component: used when fields or photos are split into 80% professional and 20% technical charges
50 Bilateral procedure (punctal plugs)
52 Reduced service (doing fields on 1 eye instead of the expected 2 eyes)
54 Surgical care only, when another physician does the post-op care
55 Post-operative management only, when another physician does the surgery
56 Pre-operative management only
76 Repeat procedure by same physician (*e.g.*, second extended ophthalmoscopy charge on 1 patient)

Notes

1. Visual fields (and in some Medicare areas, photos) cannot be charged until an interpretation is recorded in the chart.

2. Fields, photos, and sensory motor exams are billed 80% professional component, 20% technical component.

3. Contact your Medicare carrier regarding justification and documentation needed to bill extended and subsequent ophthalmoscopy.

PERSONAL MEDICAL FAMILY SOCIAL HISTORY
WITH REVIEW OF SYSTEMS — EXAMPLE

ALLERGIES

Please circle **Y** or **N** and list any allergies **you** have.

Eye Drops or other Medication Allergies.	Y N
List:____	
Itchy Eyes	Y N
Frame Materials Allergies	Y N
Hay Fever/Seasonal Allergies	Y N
Contact Lens Solution Allergies	Y N

PERSONAL MEDICAL HISTORY

Please circle **Y** if **you** have, or ever had, any of the following. Write in any medications you take.

LUNGS

Tuberculosis	Y N
Lung Cancer	Y N
Sarcoidosis	Y N
Surgery:________________________________	Y N

GASTROINTESTINAL

Asthma/Emphysema	Y N
Jaundice/Hepatitis	Y N
Ulcers/Bleeding	Y N
Hiatal Hernia	Y N
Cancer of Liver, Colon, Stomach	Y N
Surgery:________________________________	Y N

HEART

Congestive Heart Failure	Y N
Heart Murmur	Y N
Heart Attack(s)	Y N
Irregular or Fast Heart Beat	Y N
Chest Pain/Angina	Y N
High Cholesterol	Y N
Surgery:________________________________	Y N

MUSCULOSKELETAL

Degenerative Arthritis	Y N
Rheumatoid Arthritis	Y N
Polymyalgia Rheumatica	Y N
Lupus	Y N
Cancer of Bone or Muscle	Y N
Psoriasis	Y N
Surgery:________________________________	Y N

BLOOD

High Blood Pressure	Y N
Low Blood Pressure	Y N
Anemia	Y N
Sickle Cell Disease	Y N
Bleeding Disorder	Y N
Leukemia or Blood Cancer	Y N
HIV or AIDS	Y N
Other:_______________________________	Y N

NERVOUS SYSTEM

Hearing Problems	Y N
Fainting or Dizziness	Y N
Convulsions, Epilepsy, Seizures	Y N
Stroke/Paralysis	Y N
Cancer of Brain or Spinal Cord	Y N
Alzheimer's Disease	Y N
Parkinson's Disease	Y N
Other:_______________________________	Y N

ENDOCRINE

Diabetes	Y N
Cancer of Pancreas or Adrenal Glands	Y N
Thyroid Problems	Y N
Other:_______________________________	Y N

PSYCHIATRIC

Depression	Y N
Schizophrenia	Y N
Other:_______________________________	Y N

GENITOURINARY

Kidney Disease	Y N
Prostate Cancer	Y N
Cervical, Uterine, Ovarian, or Breast Cancer	Y N
Pregnant **NOW**	Y N
Other:_______________________________	Y N

EYE HISTORY

Cataract	Y N
Glaucoma	Y N
Lazy Eye or Crossed Eyes	Y N
Retinal or Macular Degeneration	Y N
Optic Nerve Problems	Y N
Night Blindness	Y N
Using Eye Drops, (list)____________________	
____________________________________	Y N

Any Eye Surgery or Injury, (list)________________

_______________________________________ Y N
List any other problem or medication
taken regularly: _______________________________

SOCIAL HISTORY
Often drink more than 2 – 3 drinks per day Y N
Do you smoke regularly? Y N
Other:_______________________________________ Y N

FAMILY HISTORY
Circle **Y** if a family member has,
or ever had, any of the following:
Glaucoma Y N
Diabetes Y N
Retinal Detachment Y N
Heart Disease Y N
Macular or Retinal Degeneration Y N
Migraine Y N
Blindness Y N
Stroke Y N

SIGNED:_______________________________________
DATE:___________

SAMPLE EXAM FORM

<table>
<tr><td colspan="2">Exam Form - example</td></tr>
<tr><td>Name____</td><td>Age___________　　　　Date___________</td></tr>
<tr><td>Last Exam____________　　Last Rx____________</td><td>Wears Rx____________</td></tr>
<tr><td>SUBJ: CC　　　　　　　　　　　　　　--></td><td>HPI</td></tr>
<tr><td>Dist. Blr　Y　N</td><td align="right">location</td></tr>
<tr><td>Near Blr　Y　N</td><td align="right">timing</td></tr>
<tr><td>Asthen.　Y　N</td><td align="right">quality</td></tr>
<tr><td>H A　　Y　N</td><td align="right">duration</td></tr>
<tr><td>Diplopia　Y　N</td><td align="right">context</td></tr>
<tr><td>Photoph.　Y　N</td><td align="right">severity</td></tr>
<tr><td>Scl. prob　Y　N</td><td align="right">mod.-factors</td></tr>
<tr><td>Eye Meds, problems:</td><td align="right">Assoc. Sx.</td></tr>
<tr><td></td><td></td></tr>
<tr><td></td><td></td></tr>
<tr><td></td><td>Tech__________</td></tr>
<tr><td>OBJECTIVE:</td><td>PD　　　　　Color　P　F　　　　Sterio</td></tr>
<tr><td>Old Rx: Glass CR39 Poly Hi Index Seg__________</td><td>BP　　　　　　Pulse　　　　　CVF　　P　F</td></tr>
<tr><td>Tint　　　　Cond　　　　　PD</td><td>TP R　　　　L　　　　　　@</td></tr>
<tr><td>PG</td><td>V 6m　　　　sc cc cl　V ph　　　J　　　sc cc</td></tr>
<tr><td>A R</td><td>Versions　S, F, No Oa　NPC</td></tr>
<tr><td>Ret</td><td>CT　Dist　　　　　　Near</td></tr>
<tr><td></td><td>VG　Lat　　　　　　V　　　　N</td></tr>
<tr><td>MR</td><td>BXC　　　　　　Demo</td></tr>
<tr><td>　　　　　　　s m d</td><td>Amp R　　　L　　　B　　　Facility G F P</td></tr>
<tr><td>K's　　　　　s m d</td><td>Pupils　　　　　DCN RRE　no APD</td></tr>
<tr><td>SL　　　wnl OD OS</td><td>Mental Status: A & O x3　wnl　　TA</td></tr>
<tr><td>Ext -Ld,Mg,Cnj,Orb,PAN　O　O</td><td>Mood and Affect　　　wnl　　TA</td></tr>
<tr><td>C -tr,epi,str,endo C&C　O　O</td><td>　　　　　　　　　　　@　　:</td></tr>
<tr><td>AC -dep,cell,flare D&Q　O　O</td><td></td></tr>
<tr><td>I　morphology　wnl　O　O</td><td></td></tr>
<tr><td>L -ac,cort,nuc,pc　wnl　O　O</td><td></td></tr>
<tr><td>DFE M & N, PMyd, Cyclo, BIO, SL, CL, Dir, Ext.</td><td></td></tr>
<tr><td>CD-R perfused, wnl　O</td><td></td></tr>
<tr><td>CD-L perfused, wnl　　O</td><td></td></tr>
<tr><td>Vas -3/4, 1/3　　O　O</td><td></td></tr>
<tr><td>Mac -flat & dry　O　O</td><td></td></tr>
<tr><td>Vit　- Clr　　O　O</td><td></td></tr>
<tr><td>Priph-flat & int.　O　O</td><td></td></tr>
<tr><td>ASSESSMENT:</td><td>PLAN:</td></tr>
<tr><td>1 RX:　CMA　CHA　M　H　Ast　Presb　Emm</td><td>1 RxSpec NoChg Opt RxCL ReplCL ReFitCL D/C CL</td></tr>
<tr><td>2 Binoc WNL</td><td>2 Monitor</td></tr>
<tr><td>3 Health WNL</td><td>3 Monitor</td></tr>
<tr><td></td><td></td></tr>
<tr><td></td><td></td></tr>
<tr><td></td><td></td></tr>
<tr><td></td><td></td></tr>
<tr><td></td><td></td></tr>
<tr><td></td><td>FINAL　R</td></tr>
<tr><td>PMFSH, Meds on Hx sheet. Review and updated</td><td>RX　　　L</td></tr>
<tr><td>Signed, Roger Filips, OD Lic 917　　　Recall__________</td><td>ADD　　　　Seg　　　　(Exp Adapt Prob)</td></tr>
</table>

MEDICAL CODING

Note—In order to simplify all of the confusing variables that need to be accounted for when coding, use the same form for all patients to give you the highest level of documentation of history. This removes the most confusing part of coding—determining the level of history obtained. See the example of Personal Medical Family Social History with Review of Systems form above. The History of Present Illness is included in the sample exam form above.

Chief Complaint (CC)—There must be a complaint that could be explained by the diagnosis you code, or the patient can be returning for you to recheck an established medical condition. Medicare does not pay for any routine or screening exams, except diabetic eye exams (250.00, 250.10, 250.20)

History of Present Illness Elements (HPI)—A minimum of 4 elements will justify up to a level 5 code.
      1) Location
      2) Timing
      3) Quality
      4) Duration
      5) Context
      6) Severity
      7) Moderating factors
      8) Associated symptoms

Personal Medical Family Social History with Review of Systems Elements (PMFSH)—See example above. Have the patient fill out this entire form at the first visit. Then have your staff update any information and record it on your new exam form. Date and initial at each follow-up visit. This is easier than trying to remember when you need to do it and when you do not need to do it.
      1) Allergies
      2) Pulmonary
      3) Cardiac
      4) Blood
      5) Endocrine
      6) Genitourinary
      7) Gastrointestinal
      8) Musculoskeletal
      9) Nervous system
      10) Psychiatric
      11) Eye history
      12) Social history
      13) Family history

Physical Exam Elements—If you are unable to do an element due to a medical reason (e.g., unable to do tonometry due to an eye infection) record why not done, and that element counts.

1) VA
2) Confrontation visual fields
3) Motility
4) Pupils
5) Mood & affect
6) Alert and oriented to person, place and time
7) IOP
8) Disk
9) Posterior segment
10) External adnexia
11) Bulbar and palpebral conjunctiva
12) Cornea
13) AC
14) Lens

Evaluation and Management (E/M) Levels—
Level 1 new (99201) requirements
A) History—any 1 HPI question
B) Exam—any 1 exam element
C) Complexity—any problem

Level 1 established (99211) requirements
A) Any visit related to a covered service, even if the patient does not see the doctor

Level 2 new (99202) requirements
A) History—any 1 HPI plus eye history
B) Exam—6 of 14 exam elements
C) Complexity—any problem

Level 2 established (99212) requirements
A) History—any 1 HPI question
B) Exam—any 1 exam element
C) Complexity—any problem

Level 3 new (99203) requirements
A) History—4 of HPI plus PMFSH
B) Exam—9 of 14 exam elements (*e.g.*, can skip DFE if mental exam is conducted)
C) Complexity
1) Diagnosis and management element options—2
2) Risk—any 1 of the following
a) 2 minor problems
b) 1 stable or chronic problem
c) 1 acute illness
d) 1 uncomplicated injury

Level 3 established (99213) requirements

A) History
  1) Any 1 of HPI
  2) Review eye questions (*e.g.*, blur, asthenopia, etc.)
      a) Exam—6 of 14 exam elements (*e.g.*, SL, VA, versions or pupils or IOP)
      b) Complexity
          1) Diagnosis and management options—2
          2) Risk—any 1 of following
              a) 2 minor problems
              b) 1 stable or chronic problem
              c) 1 acute illness
              d) 1 uncomplicated injury

Level 4 new or established (99204 or 99214)

A) History—all of the following
  1) PMFSH
  2) HPI—4 or more questions
  3) CC
B) Exam
  1) New—all procedures
  2) Established—9 of 14 exam elements (*e.g.*, can skip DFE if mental exam is conducted)
C) Complexity of decision making
  1) Number of options—**any** of the following
      a) 3 established problems or minor new problems
      b) 1 worsening established problem plus 1 stable problem
      c) Any significant new problem
  2) Amount and complexity of data—skip
  3) Risk—any **1** of following
      a) 1 chronic problem with mild worsening (*e.g.*, increased IOP)
      b) 2 stable chronic problems (*e.g.*, ARMD and cataract)
      c) 1 new diagnosis (*e.g.*, red eye)
      d) 1 acute problem with multiple symptoms (*e.g.,* facial palsy with corneal exposure)
      e) 1 acute complicated injury (*e.g.*, FB with rust ring)
      f) Prescribed a drug or did a minor procedure
      g) Cultured or did a provocative test

Level 5 new or established (99205 or 99215)

A) History—all of the following
  1) Review of systems (ROS)
  2) HPI 4 or more questions
  3) CC
  4) PMFSH
B) Exam—all 14 elements
C) Complexity of decision making—any **2** of the following
  1) Number of options—any 1 of the following
      a) New problem needing workup (*e.g.*, POAG)

     b) 1 significant new problem (*e.g.*, cataract) plus 1 other problem
     c) Worsening established problem (*e.g.*, cataract plus 2 other
       problems)
  2) Amount and complexity of data—review and summarize any 1 of
    the following
     a) Get old records
     b) Call previous doctor
     c) Get history from a family member or other care giver
  3) Risk—**either** of the following
     a) Threat to life or eye (*e.g.*, closed angle, amaurosis fugax,
       giant cell arteritis, hot iritis, ulcer, nerve swelling, retinal hole,
       other retinal problems)
     b) Prescribe multiple drugs with toxicity

Time—Time is a factor only if the total face-to-face doctor time spent with the patient exceeds the number of minutes listed below, AND over half of the time is spent in counseling or coordination of care. Then, the time spent with the patient is the only factor to consider when choosing a billing level. Record total time and counseling/coordination time in record.

New patient
  Level 1, 10 min
  Level 2, 20 min
  Level 3, 30 min
  Level 4, 45 min
  Level 5, 60 min

Established patient
  Level 1, 5 min
  Level 2, 10 min
  Level 3, 15 min
  Level 4, 25 min
  Level 5, 40 min

Comprehensive vision exam 92004 or 92014
A) History—PMFSH
B) Exam—8 of 14 exam elements
C) Complexity—skip
D) Risk—initiation of diagnosis or treatment, any 1 of the following
    ("Monitor" or continuing same Tx not enough)
  1) Scheduling diagnostic testing
  2) Referring for consultation
  3) Prescribing for glasses with a 2-line improvement in VA if the Rx
    change is due to a medical condition such as cataract or diabetes
  4) Prescribing a new therapy

DIOPTER CONVERSION TABLE

Diopters Converted into Millimeters

D	mm	D	mm	D	mm	D	mm	D	mm	D	mm	D	mm	D	mm
20.00	16.88	36.00	9.38	39.00	8.65	42.00	8.04	45.00	7.50	48.00	7.03	51.00	6.62	54.00	6.25
22.00	15.34	36.12	9.34	39.12	8.63	42.12	8.01	45.12	7.48	48.12	7.01	51.12	6.60	54.12	6.24
24.00	14.06	36.25	9.31	39.25	8.60	42.25	7.99	45.25	7.46	48.25	6.99	51.25	6.59	54.25	6.22
26.00	12.98	36.37	9.28	39.37	8.57	42.37	7.97	45.37	7.44	48.37	6.98	51.37	6.57	54.37	6.21
27.00	12.50	36.50	9.25	39.50	8.54	42.50	7.94	45.50	7.42	48.50	6.96	51.50	6.55	54.50	6.19
28.00	12.05	36.62	9.22	39.62	8.52	42.62	7.92	45.62	7.40	48.62	6.94	51.62	6.54	54.62	6.18
29.00	11.64	36.75	9.18	39.75	8.49	42.75	7.89	45.75	7.38	48.75	6.92	51.75	6.52	54.75	6.16
29.50	11.44	36.87	9.15	39.87	8.47	42.87	7.87	45.87	7.36	48.87	6.91	51.87	6.51	54.87	6.15
30.00	11.25	37.00	9.12	40.00	8.44	43.00	7.85	46.00	7.34	49.00	6.89	52.00	6.49	55.00	6.14
30.50	11.07	37.12	9.09	40.12	8.41	43.12	7.83	46.12	7.32	49.12	6.87	52.12	6.48	55.12	6.12
31.00	10.89	37.25	9.06	40.25	8.39	43.25	7.80	46.25	7.30	49.25	6.85	52.25	6.46	55.25	6.11
31.50	10.71	37.37	9.03	40.37	8.36	43.37	7.78	46.37	7.25	49.37	6.84	52.37	6.44	55.37	6.10
32.00	10.55	37.50	9.00	40.50	8.33	43.50	7.76	46.50	7.26	49.50	6.82	52.50	6.43	55.50	6.08
32.50	10.39	37.62	8.97	40.62	8.31	43.62	7.74	46.62	7.24	49.62	6.80	52.62	6.41	55.62	6.07
33.00	10.23	37.75	8.94	40.75	8.28	43.75	7.71	46.75	7.22	49.75	6.78	52.75	6.40	55.75	6.05
33.50	10.08	37.87	8.91	40.87	8.26	43.87	7.69	46.87	7.20	49.87	6.77	52.87	6.38	55.87	6.04
34.00	9.93	38.00	8.88	41.00	8.23	44.00	7.67	47.00	7.18	50.00	6.75	53.00	6.37	56.00	6.03
34.25	9.85	38.12	8.85	41.12	8.21	44.12	7.65	47.12	7.16	50.12	6.73	53.12	6.35	56.50	5.97
34.50	9.78	38.25	8.82	41.25	8.18	44.25	7.63	47.25	7.14	50.25	6.72	53.25	6.34	57.00	5.92
34.75	9.71	38.37	8.80	41.37	8.16	44.37	7.61	47.37	7.12	50.37	6.70	53.37	6.32	57.50	5.87
35.00	9.64	38.50	8.77	41.50	8.13	44.50	7.58	47.50	7.11	50.50	6.68	53.50	6.31	58.00	5.82
35.25	9.57	38.62	8.74	41.62	8.11	44.62	7.56	47.62	7.09	50.62	6.67	53.62	6.29	58.50	5.77
35.50	9.51	38.75	8.71	41.75	8.08	44.75	7.54	47.75	7.07	50.75	6.65	53.75	6.28	59.00	5.72
35.75	9.44	38.87	8.68	41.87	8.06	44.87	7.52	47.87	7.05	50.87	6.63	53.87	6.27	60.00	5.63

VERTEX CONVERSION TABLE

Spectacle Lens Power	Plus Lenses				Minus Lenses			
	8	10	12	14	8	10	12	14
4.00	4.12	4.12	4.25	4.25	3.87	3.87	3.87	3.75
4.50	4.62	4.75	4.75	4.75	4.37	4.25	4.25	4.25
5.00	5.25	5.25	5.25	5.37	4.75	4.75	4.75	4.62
5.50	5.75	5.75	5.87	6.00	5.25	5.25	5.12	5.12
6.00	6.25	6.37	6.50	6.50	5.75	5.62	5.62	5.50
6.50	6.87	7.00	7.00	7.12	6.12	6.12	6.00	6.00
7.00	7.37	7.50	7.62	7.75	6.62	6.50	6.50	6.37
7.50	8.00	8.12	8.25	8.37	7.12	7.00	3.87	6.75
8.00	8.50	8.75	8.87	9.00	7.50	7.37	7.25	7.25
8.50	9.12	9.25	9.50	9.62	8.00	7.87	7.75	7.62
9.00	9.75	9.87	10.12	10.37	8.37	8.25	8.12	8.00
9.50	10.25	10.50	10.75	11.00	8.87	8.62	8.50	8.37
10.00	10.87	11.12	11.37	11.62	9.25	9.12	8.87	8.75
10.50	11.50	11.75	12.00	12.25	9.62	9.50	9.37	9.12
11.00	12.00	12.37	12.75	13.00	10.12	9.87	9.75	9.50
11.50	12.62	13.00	13.37	13.75	10.50	10.37	10.12	9.87
12.00	13.25	13.62	14.00	14.50	11.00	10.75	10.50	10.25
12.50	13.87	14.25	14.75	15.25	11.37	11.12	10.87	10.62
13.00	14.50	15.00	15.50	16.00	11.75	11.50	11.25	11.00
13.50	15.12	15.62	16.12	16.62	12.25	11.87	11.62	11.37
14.00	15.75	16.25	16.75	17.50	12.62	12.25	12.00	11.75
14.50	16.50	17.00	17.50	18.25	13.00	12.62	12.37	12.00
15.00	17.00	17.75	18.25	19.00	13.37	13.00	12.75	12.37
15.50	17.75	18.25	19.00	19.75	13.75	13.50	13.00	12.75
16.00	18.25	19.00	19.75	20.50	14.25	13.75	13.50	13.00
16.50	19.00	19.75	20.50	21.50	14.50	14.12	13.75	13.50
17.00	19.75	20.50	21.50	22.25	15.00	14.50	14.12	13.75
17.50	20.50	21.25	22.25	23.25	15.37	14.87	14.50	14.00
18.00	21.00	22.00	23.00	24.00	15.75	15.25	14.75	14.37
18.50	21.75	22.75	23.75	25.00	16.12	15.62	15.12	14.75
19.00	22.50	23.50	24.75	26.00	16.50	16.00	15.50	15.00

INDEX

A

Abducens 97, 108
Abrasions 7, 20, 22, 31, 32, 73
Acanthamoeba 31
Accommodative dysfunction, *see* Chap. 30 (149–152)
Acebutolol 15
Acetazolamide 10, 14
Acne rosacea 8
ACUTE ANGLE CLOSURE GLAUCOMA (Chap. 7) 49–50
Acyclovir 8, 32, 33
Adalat 15
Adie's tonic pupil 100, 101
ADVANCED INTERPRETATION OF HUMPHREY VISUAL FIELDS IN GLAUCOMA (Chap. 9) 63–68
Advil 11
Afferent pupillary defect 103, 107, 111, 113
AGE RELATED MACULAR DEGENERATION (Chap. 10) 69–70
Aldactone 14
Alkali burns 20, 21
Allegra 13
Allergic conjunctivitis 28
Allergy
    Alphagan 58
    anti-allergy drops 2
    aspirin 11
    benadryl 10
    conjunctivitis 28
    glaucoma 59
    history 181, 185
    NSAID 11
    opioid 11
    pediatric eye exam 130
    penicillin 5–8
    seasonal 9
    steroid drops 1
    sulfa 7, 10, 14
    uveitis 45
Alpha-glucosidase inhibitors 72
Alphagan 3, 58, 59
Altace 16
Amaurosis fugax 94, 188
Amiodarone 15
Amlodipine 15
Amoxicillin 5, 6
Ampicillin 5
Analgesia 2
Angina 15, 16, 187
Angiotensin converting enzyme (ACE) inhibitors 16, 41
Anisocoria 21, 22, 95, 99, 100, 101
Ankylosing spondylitis 41
Anterior chamber 20

Antiarrhythmics 15
Antinuclear antibody (ANA) 41, 42
Antianginals 14
Antibiotics
    broad spectrum 23
    continue 20
    discontinue 122
    drops 1
    fortified 30, 31
    ointment 1, 2
    recommendations 5
    topical 1, 61, 119, 121
Antihistamines 8, 9, 13
Antivirals 1, 8, 33
Anxiety 16
APPENDIX 157–191
Aqueous 14, 16, 36, 38, 39, 53
Argon laser trabeculoplasty (ALT) 36, 60
Argyll Robertson syndrome 100
Arrhythmia 15, 16
Arteritis 89, 90, 91, 94, 97
Artery 85
Arthritis
    history 181
    orals for eyecare 6, 11
    side effects, medications 13
    uveitis 40–42, 45
Artificial tears 2
Aspirin
    beta blockers 15
    blood thinners 16
    contraindications, orals for eyecare 10, 11
    diabetes 76
    injuries 23
    neovascular sudden vision loss 91
    red eye miscellaneous 27
    side effects, medications 15, 16, 17
    sudden monocular vision loss 86, 88
Asthma 16, 181
Atenolol 15
Atropine 3, 20, 23, 32, 38
Augmentin 5, 6
Avonex 94
Azopt 3, 10, 49, 58

B

Bacitracin 1, 21, 25, 32
Background diabetic retinopathy (BDR) 73
Bacterial conjunctivitis 28
Bacterial keratitis 31
Bactrim 5, 7
Benazepril 16
Beta blockers 3, 15, 16, 49, 51, 58
Betadine 31
Betaxolol 15
Biaxin 5, 7

Amsler Grid

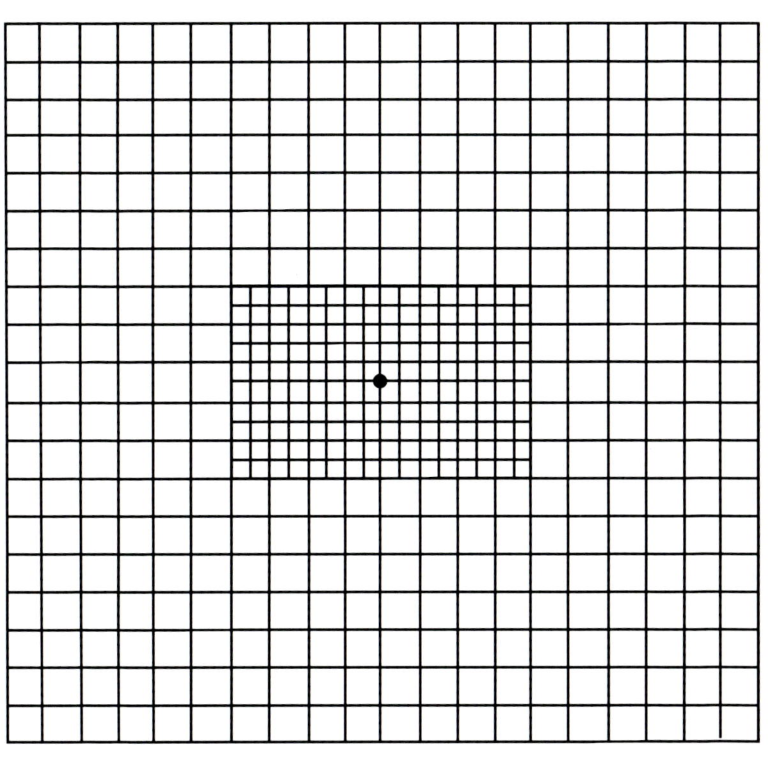

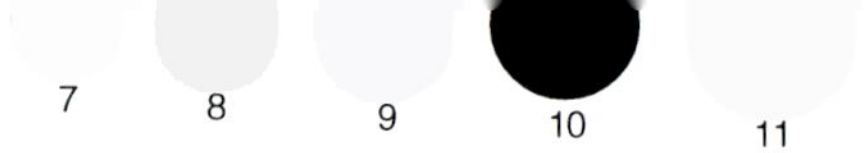

3   4   5   6   7   8   9   10   11   mm

400   E B F Z

200   Z C O T

150   C B Y S

100   F H O D

80   P H T C

60   D A O F

50   E G N D H

40   F Z V O E

30   O F L C T

A P E O T F

20   T Z V E C L

F O F Z E C

AMSLER GRID

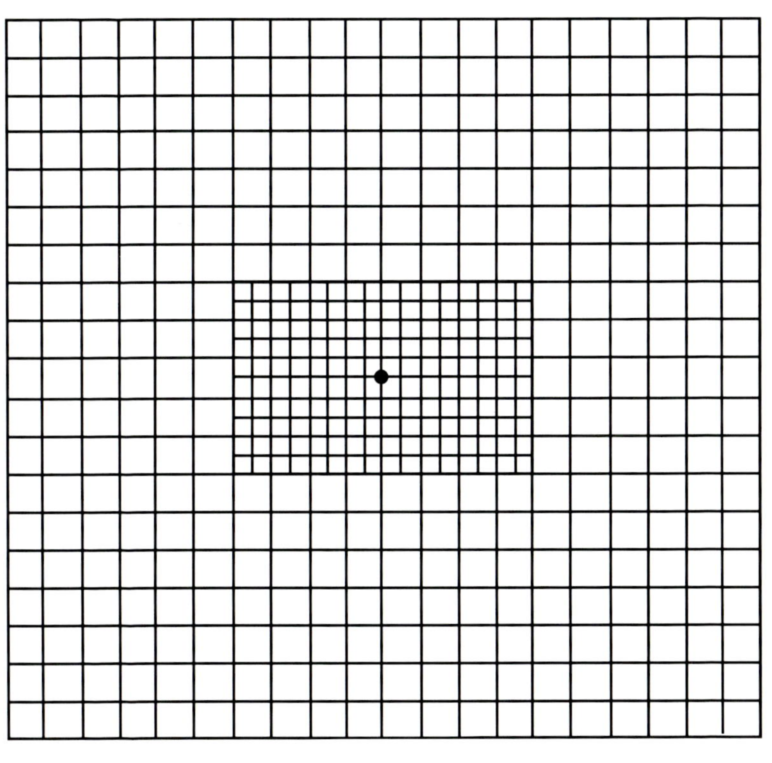

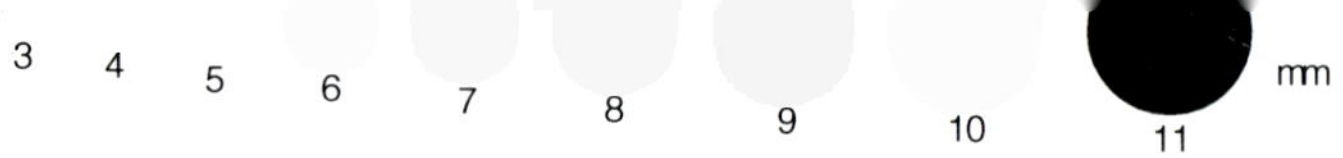

3 4 5 6 7 8 9 10 11 mm

400 E B F Z

200 Z C O T

150 C B Y S

100 F H O D

80 P H T C

60 D A O F

50 E G N D H

40 F Z V O E

30 O F L C T

A P E O T F

20 T Z V E C L

F O P Z E C